NILS CHRISTIE

Limits to Pain

MARTIN ROBERTSON · OXFORD

© Universitetsforlaget 1981

Published simultaneously in Norway by Universitetsforlaget
and in the United Kingdom by Martin Robertson & Company Ltd.

First published in the United Kingdom in 1982 by
Martin Robertson & Company Ltd.,
108 Cowley Road, Oxford OX4 1JF.

British Library Cataloguing in Publication Data
Christie, Nils
    Limits to pain.
    1.   Crime and criminals — Social aspects
    2.   Punishment — Social aspects
    I.   Title
    364   HV6025

    ISBN 0-85520-476-1
    ISBN 0-85520-475-3 Pbk

Cover design by Bruno Oldani
Printed in Norway by Dreyer Aksjeselskap, Stavanger

Preface

The major ideas in this little book are simple.

The reasoning is as follows: imposing punishment within the institution of law means the inflicting of pain, intended as pain. This is an activity which often comes in dissonance to esteemed values such as kindness and forgiveness. To reconcile these incompatibilities, attempts are sometimes made to hide the basic character of punishment. In cases where hiding is not possible, all sorts of reasons for intentional infliction of pain are given. One major effort in what follows is to describe, expose, and evaluate major features of these attempts, and to relate them to general social conditions.

None of the attempts to cope with the intended pain seems, however, to be quite satisfactory. Attempts to change the law-breaker create problems of justice. Attempts to inflict only a just measure of pain create rigid systems insensitive to individual needs. It is as if societies in their struggle with penal theories and practices oscillate between attempts to solve some unsolvable dilemmas.

My own view is that the time is now ripe to bring these oscillatory moves to an end by describing their futility and by taking a moral stand in favour of creating severe restrictions on the use of man-made pain as a means of social control. On the basis of experience from social systems with a minimal use of pain, some general conditions for a low level of pain infliction are extracted.

If pain is to be applied, it has to be pain without a manipulative purpose and in a social form resembling that which is used when people are in deep sorrow. This might lead to a situation where punishment for crime evaporated. Where that happened, basic features of the State would also have evaporated. Formulated as an ideal, this situation might be just as valuable to make explicit and to keep in mind as situations where kindness and humanity reign – ideals never to be reached, but something to stretch towards.

I am grateful to so many friends and colleagues who have helped. All Souls College, Oxford, functioned as a sanctuary during parts of the work, and Roger Hood and Adam Podgorecki gave friendship and advice. Louk Hulsman and Herman Bianchi have acted as important sources of inspiration from Holland. Rick Abel, Kettil Bruun, Andrew von Hirsch, and Stan Wheeler have offered helpful criticism of a first draft of the manuscript. Grants from the German Marshall Foundation and the Scandinavian Research Council for Criminology provided the opportunity for a meeting in June 1980 where examples of participatory justice were thoroughly discussed.

Nonetheless, it is a book from Scandinavia. By writing in a foreign language, one comes in a way closer to home. From here I have most of my experiences. And here I receive, year after year, generous criticism and encouragement. For this particular manuscript, I have received valuable help from Vigdis and Lindis Charlotte Christie, Tove Stang Dahl, Kjersti Ericsson, Sturla Falck, Hedda Giertsen, Cecilie Høigård, Per Ole Johansen, Leif Petter Olaussen, Annika Snare, Per Stangeland and Dag Østerberg. I have not always listened to my advisers, so none of them are responsible for defects in the final product.

Oslo, March 1981
Nils Christie

Table of contents

Chapter 1. On Pain

This is a book about pain. But I do not quite know what pain is, or how to graduate it. Literature is full of heroes so great that pain becomes small, or cowards so small that almost everything becomes pain. To grasp the essence of pain, one would have to understand the core of the good as well as the evil. I refrain from the attempt.

Those who look at penal history as stages in progress might argue that I refrain too fast. They would see developments, a gradual decrease in pain, which would make ranking possible. From Foucault's (1975) opening description of the gruesome public execution of Damiens in 1757, through the Norwegian Parliamentary invention in 1815 of a tariff converting branding and cutting off limbs into terms of imprisonment – ten years for a hand – does it not exemplify reduction in pain? From slaveries and workhouses with their uncontrolled abuses, to well-ordered penitentiaries, is that not progress? From whipping for disobedience to loss of privileges? From the old smelling stone castles to single rooms with hot and cold water, – does that not exemplify reduction in pain?

I just do not know. Each form would have to be evaluated according to its own time, by those receiving the pain, in the framework of their usual life and other people's usual life, and in the light of what they saw as their sins. I do not see how a scale could be established.

Protagonists of hard-data science might also argue that I refrain too fast. We can certainly measure how the nerves are distributed in the body. Or we can standardize situations and persons, and find out what they report as most painful.

We can, and the more so the closer we move towards the physiology of the phenomena. But at the same time, the closer we move towards nerve-centres and standardized situations, the further we move *away* from those social, ethical, and religious elements that seem able to neutralize what ought to have been severe pain, or to aggravate minor pain. Guards in concentration camps (Christie 1972) described with surprise how prisoners reacted more to minor than to major violence. "They cried, as children, if receiving a small cuff. But it was as if they did not react at all if very severely beaten, or if friends were killed." Jacques Lusseyran (1963) is very close to saying that he enjoyed life in the concentration camp of Buchenwald. He was continuously close to extinction. Of the 2 000 on his train from France, 30 survived. He had to use his hand to find his way and discriminate between the dead and the half-dead in the infirmary. He was blind from childhood. Social anthropology has accounts of villagers singing outside an offender's house. It proves sufficiently painful to drive the offender to death.

For these and other reasons, this book will not discuss what pain is, whether certain pains are greater than other, or whether pain on earth has decreased or increased. Those questions are greater than social science. But what I can do, and will, is to describe some *acts* intended as punishments and also some acts very similar to those intended as punishment. I will describe some *forms* used when decisions on such acts are made. And I will *evaluate* acts as well as forms.

Moralism within our areas has for some years been an attitude or even a term associated with protagonists for law and order and severe penal sanctions, while their opponents were seen as floating in a sort of value-free vacuum. Let it therefore be completely clear that I am also a moralist. Worse: I am a moral imperialist. One of my basic premises will be that it is right to strive for a reduction of man-inflicted pain on earth. I can very well see objections to this position.

Pain makes people grow. They become more mature – twice born – receive deeper insights, experience more joy if pain fades, and according to some belief-systems they come closer to God or Heaven. Some among us might have experienced some of these benefits. But we have also experienced the opposite: Pain which brings growth to a stop, pain which retards, pain which makes people evil. In any case: I cannot imagine a position where I should strive for an increase of man-inflicted pain on earth. Nor can I see any good reason to believe that the recent level of pain-infliction is just the right or natural one. And since the matter is important, and I feel compelled to make a choice, I see no other defensible position than to strive for pain-reduction.

One of the rules would then be: If in doubt, do not pain. Another rule would be: Inflict as little pain as possible. Look for alternatives to punishments, not only alternative punishments. It is often not necessary to react; the offender as well as the surroundings know it was wrong. Much deviance is expressive, a clumsy attempt to say something. Let the crime then become a starting point for a real dialogue, and not for an equally clumsy answer in the form of a spoonful of pain. Social systems must be constructed so that a dialogue can take place. Furthermore: Some systems are created in ways that make it natural to perceive many acts as crime. Others are constructed in ways where the same acts are more easily seen as expressions of conflicting interests. To reduce man-inflicted pain, one should encourage construction of the latter type of systems. In the simplification needed here, and well aware that complex matters are shelved, my position can be condensed into views that social systems ought to be constructed in ways that reduce to a minimum the perceived need for infliction of pain for the purpose of social control. Sorrow is inevitable, but not hell created by man.

Chapter 2. The Shield of Words

The seriousness of the core phenomena within penal law is easily forgotten.

If an employee in a funeral bureau allowed himself to become involved with all the sorrow he encountered, if he took it on and in himself, he would soon have to change his occupation. The same is probably the case for those among us who work in, or are closely connected with, the penal law system. The questions confronting us are difficult to live with. We survive by turning the work into routine, by engaging in only small bits of the totality at a time, and by distancing ourselves from the client, particularly from the client's experience of her or his own situation.

Words are a good means of disguising the character of our activities. Funeral agencies have a vocabulary perfectly suited to survival. The deceased has "gone to rest" or to "sleep", the sufferings have ceased, the body is made beautiful again, and in the USA, the farewell party is arranged by professionals in a funeral home.

We do the same thing within the crime-control system and its surroundings. How characteristic, is it not, that I have already in this chapter used the word "client" twice instead of, as a minimum, "the person to be punished". "Client" is a convenient term, in olden times meaning "dependent", often used for a person to whom we offer service or help. Inside prisons, at least in my part of the world, he is called "inmate", not "prisoner". His room in the prison is called just that: "room", not "cell". If he misbehaves, he might be offered "single-room-treatment". In practice this might mean days of isolation in a cell stripped of furniture. Most of the personnel within prisons in my country are called *"betjent"*, which means one who serves. They are not called "guards". We are, however, rather moderate in the use of euphemisms at the top level of the Norwegian prison system. We call prison-directors what they are: "prison-directors"; we likewise call the highest administrative body the "prison-board". In Sweden they call the top level "Kriminal*vård*-styrelsen". *"Vård"* gives associations of caretaking. The Danish director for the whole system is called the director for the crime-*"forsorg"*, which is the word we use for those in need of care: the sick, the old, the very poor, the small children who have nobody else to come to. General use of the word *"forsorg"* was abandoned when social security was introduced and to a large extent medicalized. So, now the term has become available for new purposes, such as a title for the director of the system in charge of delivering penal sanctions.

What sort of words ought we to opt for?

There are certainly many kind thoughts behind the kind words. Prisoners might feel better were they not constantly reminded of their status by being called "prisoners", placed in "cells", transferred to "special punishments cells", watched by "guards", and directed by "prison directors". Maybe they would feel less stigmatized. Maybe they would receive more service and help if the system were called *"forsorg"* instead of "prison". Maybe kind words create a kind world. What makes me wonder whether there is not more to it than mere kindness is the easy acceptance of these kind words among those in authority. It is not those in sorrow who put a ban on expressing grief. It is society, assisted by the funeral directors. As Geoffrey Gorer (1965) has pointed out: In our types of societies there exists a strong taboo against expressing severe sorrow and grief. Suffering is to be expressed in a controlled form, and not for long. This is supposed to be best for those closest to death and misery. Certainly it is good for those not so close.

Through language and ceremony, grief has vanished from public life. But so have also the pains of punishment. When we used flogging, cutting off parts of the body, or killing as punishment, the suffering was more obvious (except for the wicked group who tricked the authorities into executing them and were thereby spared the most sinful act of committing suicide). Heavy chains symbolized the degradation. It was a clear-cut picture of sorrow and misery. Today, some prisons look like modern motels, other like boarding-schools. Decent food, work or education, males and females in the same unit in sinful Denmark, conjugal visits in Sweden, it all looks like a vacation at the tax-payers' expense.

In line with this, the phenomenon of pain and suffering has close to evaporated, even in text-books on penal law. Most texts make it clear that punishment is an evil intended as an evil. But beyond this, modern texts do not go much further. Compared to the enormous wealth of detail and subtle distinctions usually offered in these text-books, there exists a remarkable reservation among recent authors when it comes to a description of the core phenomena, the penalties. How the punishments hurt, how it feels, the suffering and the sorrow, these are elements most often completely lacking in the texts. And they are not lacking just by oversight, as one discovers if one challenges penal law writers on their sterile coverage of the core phenomena of their trade and suggests that they ought to become a bit more concrete in their writing. The word penal is closely related to pain. This is more obvious in the language tradition of English and French than in the German/Scandinavian one, where we talk about "*Strafferett*" or "*Straf-recht*", that is "punishment law". But in both language traditions considerable turmoil is created if it is suggested that the basic law should be called a "pain-law". I have done it, so I know. The penal law

15

professors do most definitely not like to be designated "pain-law" professors. The judges do not like to sentence people to pain. Their preference is to sentence them to various "measures". The receiving institutions do not like to be regarded or to regard themselves, as "pain-inflicting" institutions. Still, such a terminology would actually present a very precise message: punishment as administered by the penal law system is the conscious inflicting of pain. Those who are punished are supposed to suffer. If they by and large enjoyed it, we would change the method. It is intended within penal institutions that those at the receiving end shall get something that makes them unhappy, something that hurts.

Crime control has become a clean, hygienic operation. Pain and suffering have vanished from the text-books and from the applied labels. But of course not from the experience of those punished. The targets for penal action are just as they used to be: scared, ashamed, unhappy. Sometimes hidden behind a rough facade, but one which is easily penetrated, as exemplified in many studies. Martha Baum shows in detail how "little old men" become very little when confronted with the fact that they were not to go home to mother (in Wheeler 1968). Cohen and Taylor (1972) describe techniques for "psychological survival". Such techniques are not necessary if suffering does not exist. The whole book is one single sad tale of the successes of those who intended to create suffering in other people. So is also Sykes' (1958) description of what he rightly calls "the pains of imprisonment". And that is what is conveyed in the prisoners' own words. A man just out of one of Castro's prisons describes his destiny in an interview with Inger Holt-Seeland in the Danish newspaper *Information* (11 December 1979). He measures time through changes in those visiting him:

I will make an attempt to give you a sort of film version of how time is passing for the prisoner. Try to imagine the first year, when the visits were

16

coloured by the children. They came, running ahead, followed by some young, beautiful women . . . they moved fast . . . behind them, more slowly, came parents, siblings, parents-in-law, loaded with heavy bags. Some years later, things have changed. Now some young people come first – they are not children any more, they are youngsters, 12, 13 and 14 years, then follow what now are middle-aged women in their thirties, with different movements, with different expressions on their faces . . . and those who were 40 or 50 are now 60 or . . ., they now come far behind, slowly . . . and just as the character of the visit changes so do their clothes, people are wearing darker clothes, use fewer gestures, the high voices are gone, the jokes are gone, the anecdotes and the stories are gone, only the essentials are talked about. The visit becomes sadder, fewer words are spoken, joy has left . . . And as for the prisoners, their heads have become white, their faces wrinkled, their teeth are going . . .

This man spent 18 years behind the walls. So, in Scandinavia we have an easy way out. We can tell ourselves that "this does not happen here", "not that long", "not long at all, for the great majority". Which is all correct. But only up to a point.

If we take the trouble to penetrate the facades of Scandinavian design, we meet these supposed vacationers who happen to be as miserable in the few cases of modern Scandinavian design, as they were reported to be in the old Philadelphia-type prisons. How could it be otherwise? Prisoners share most of ordinary peoples' values. They are placed before the judge and inside walls as a consequence of acts they are supposed to be ashamed of. If they are not ashamed of the acts, they are at least ashamed of being in the situation. And if not ashamed, at least filled with sadness by the simple fact that life is passing by without their participation.

While writing this, a characteristic illustration of what penal law professors do not cover in their texts arrived in my mail. The journal *Nordisk medisin* (1980) devotes most of its March issue to the question of pain. The whole front cover is a picture of a face in agony, and the content is devoted to the relief of pain. The editorial (Lindblom 1980, p. 75) says:

To stimulate and coordinate research on pain, and to improve teaching on the results of this research, a new interdisciplinary organization has been created. It has been named International Association for the Study of Pain.

As the result of US-experience, new ways of handling severe cases of pain have been attempted, particularly chronic conditions where treatment for the cause of pain is not possible. Interdisciplinary treatment of pain in the form of pain-clinics of the type that exist in USA, England and certain other European countries has however still not come into being in Scandinavia . . .

The research is interdisciplinary. One wonders what would happen if penal experts were included. Would they then compare notes, and try to construct all the other parties' negations? Penologists might thereby learn more efficient ways of creating pain, doctors more efficient ways to prevent it.

But of course, penologists in our cultures would not opt for membership in the Interdisciplinary Association for the Study of Pain. They would become provoked and angry even by the mere suggestion. Attendance would make clear what is now blurred. There might be only small problems in delivering pain in societies where pain is the explicit destiny for most people: pain on Earth, pain in Hell. (Even though the ambiguous status of the hangman indicated that the problems back in time were not insignificant.) But that society is not ours. We have abolished Hell, and have pain-reduction on earth as one of the major goals. In such a society it is difficult to let people suffer intentionally.

Still we do it. We inflict intended pain. But we do not like it. Our choice of neutralizing words deceives us; the law professors' bleak description of the qualities of the intended sufferings indicates the same. We do not like the activity because intentionally causing pain is in grave dissonance with other basic activities in our society.

In this book I often apply the words "pain delivery". But I have had to make a considerable effort to preserve that formulation from extinction. My kind and highly qualified adviser in the subtleties of the English language has insisted that the term does not exist. Pain delivery, it sounds like milk delivery. Dreadful. My point has been the opposite: It sounds like milk delivery. Perfect. This captures exactly what I want to convey. If pain delivery is not a concept in Oxford English, it ought to become one. Pain delivery is the concept for what in our time has developed into a calm, efficient, hygienic operation. Seen from the perspective of those delivering the service, it is not first and foremost drama, tragedy, intense sufferings. Infliction of pain is in dissonance with some major ideals, but can be carried out in an innocent, somnambulistic insulation from the value conflict. The pains of punishments are left to the receivers. Through the choice of words, working routines, division of labour and repetition, the whole thing has become the delivery of a commodity.

Chapter 3. Treatment for Crime

3.1. From alcohol to dangerousness

Scandinavians have severe problems with alcohol. We do not consume great quantities according to international standards, but we consume it in situations and ways that enable drinkers to evade the usual forms of social control. It will therefore be easily understood that drinking, and control of drinking, have been topics of focal concern within our societies. It has been an important and difficult problem: important through the many and highly visible signs of misery. Difficult because we want to get rid of the problem, but not of the alcohol. Therefore we could not, as with heroin for example, outlaw the whole substance. Vis-à-vis most drugs we apply an official policy of teetotalism. Except in situations governed by medicine-men we decree the drugs unsuitable for everybody. When it comes to alcohol, that type of control seems impossible. Here we operate with the idea that the problems are not in the substance, alcohol, but in certain categories of users. We have of course also a vast number of rules and regulations concerning the sale and serving of alcohol. But in addition to the partial control of the substance, we do attempt to control some categories of those who cannot hold their liquor.

It was particularly the skid-row population we made the first attempts to control. Drunken people in the streets were a distasteful and unaesthetic nuisance. Teetotallers used them as pedagogical examples, the alcohol users found them embarrassing. Drunkards therefore should be kept out of circulation. It was not easy, however, to regard their behaviour as so disgusting that they deserved a punishment which would keep them away for a sufficiently long time to create a real improvement in the renovation of the streets.

But what could not justly be done in the name of punishment could not be objected to if it were carried out as treatment. Treatment might also hurt. But so many a cure hurts. And this pain is not intended as pain. It is intended as a cure. Pain becomes thus unavoidable, but ethically acceptable. The idea was formulated at a major meeting of the Norwegian Association for Criminal Policy in 1893, and it took only a few years until a law based on this principle was passed in Parliament. The law authorized the crime-control system to put people away for treatment if they had been arrested several times for drunkenness in the street. Instead of fines for drunkenness, they should, since they were not deterred by the fines, receive a long period of treatment. The original idea was that the period for which people should be put away would be completely indeterminate. At the last minute, however, a limit of four years was decided upon. This was to be spent in what turned out to be the most severe prison in the country, situated on a flat and dull piece of land so windy that, according to one of the directors, the hens had to be tied to the ground so as not to be blown away. Recidivists were given another four years, and then followed as many four-year periods as needed, until the cure was completed.

Similar measures were also installed in Sweden and Finland but not in Denmark. Denmark has always coped with alcohol and alcohol-problems in ways more similar to those common in Central Europe. In Finland the measure was particularly useful, because it was combined with an arrangement whereby those incarcerated could apply for deportation to Siberia instead. Many did.

But not all sickness can be cured. The concept of the ''non-treatable'' is the logical extension of ideas of treatment.

Some sick people cannot be helped back into ordinary life. They have to be kept, as old people in nursing homes, or as the completely disabled in their special units. It would not be fair to expect complete success within the crime-control system either. Therefore, this system would also be in need of more permanent units for the hard core, particularly since this system would also be confronted with people diagnosed as *dangerous criminals*. Again, it might be experienced as painful to live in such an institution. But so was also often the fate of the old or permanently disabled. And in the particular case of the dangerous criminals, pains of potential victims were prevented.

This whole development reached a climax in Sweden just after the Second World War. A penal law committee proposed the complete abolition of the old penal law and of the concept of punishment. Sweden should have a law of "measures" for social defence, not of punishments. The proposition was defeated.

3.2. The great explorers

Last century was the age of voyages of discovery. Livingstone explored Africa for the white man, sociologists were investigating the situation of the lower classes in the European cities. Machines grew bigger and more powerful. They demanded more hard-working hands in the towns and fewer in the country. It became more difficult to control the masses in the towns. The operators of the machines drew physically nearer and yet, at the same time, they became more remote. August Strindberg, describing the Stockholm of the last century (The Maid-Servant's Son 1878), tells us how the civil servant, the burgher, the worker and the whore at one time lived together in the same building, though not in similar apartments. Gradually, however, their ways parted. Valen-Senstad (1953) describes how in Oslo no policeman in his right mind ventured alone into Vaterland. It was like Harlem today, enemy territory, or at any rate the territory of the aliens.

Working in Italy at that time was a young military doctor, Cesare Lombroso. He himself tells of the breakthrough he made on one occasion in the 1860's.

Suddenly, one morning on a gloomy day in December, I found in the skull of a brigand a very long series of atavistic abnormalities . . . analogous to those that are found in inferior vertebrates. At the sight of these strange abnormalities, – as an extensive plain is lit up by a glowing horizon – I realized that the problem of the nature and generation of criminals was resolved for me. (Radzinowicz 1966, p. 29).

Recently questions have been raised as to the nature of these "brigands". Were they plain criminals, robbers? Or were they farmer-rebels? Was the question of the nature and cause of criminality solved on the basis of the skull of a political enemy? In any case: the causes of crime were firmly placed inside the body. Criminals were different from most other people. And they had to be met with scientific methods. They had to be dealt with either through internment or by treatment, in accordance with the needs of the particular criminal.

Lombroso was the flagship. In his wake came Ferri in Italy, von Liszt in Germany, Bernhard Getz in Scandinavia – and then all the special regulations and measures relating to the particular circumstances of the individual lawbreaker. We acquired preventive detention, remand in custody, indeterminate sentences and experts to decide the moment of discharge, institutions for psychopaths and special institutions for alcoholics. The liberal state was not all that liberal when it came to the establishment of the external conditions for the free flow of economic entrepreneurship. Roads, railroads and regulating the poor became essential. An army of experts evolved. Deviance control became essential for industrial development. The intellectual foundations for this way of thinking were established in the nineteenth century. Tove Stang Dahl describes this development in two important works (1977, 1978). Ignatieff (1978, p. 215) comes to the same conclusions: "The intensification of Labour discipline went hand in hand in hand with the elaboration of the freedom of a market in Labour, ..."

3.3. The downfall of an empire

During the last ten years, these measures have nearly all vanished.[1]

The skid-row population was allowed to remain on the streets in my country from 1970. Special measures against psychopaths are increasingly going out of fashion. Denmark and Finland have dropped the system altogether, Norway and Sweden are soon to follow. Borstal institutions and special youth prisons have been abolished everywhere, except in Sweden. The remaining major exception has to do with the so-called "dangerous criminal". Denmark had 20 persons classified as such in 1978, Finland 9. Norway will probably find a solution corresponding to Finland's when we abolish special measures against psychopaths. A recent Swedish committee has proposed to drop the category "equal to insanity". By and large we are back to a system with definite sentences decided by the courts.

To a large extent, this was bound to happen. First: The hypocrisy of the system soon became transparent. One study after another indicated that the treatment centres for criminals were not hospitals after all. They were suspiciously

[1] The story of the heyday and later demise of "treatment for crime" has been told by so many and in so much detail, that I can make my coverage very short.
Some early Scandinavian works with a critique of treatment ideology and its results can be found in Aubert (1958), Christie (1960 a and b), Aubert and Mathiesen (1962), Børjeson (1966), Eriksson (1967), Anttila (1967) and Bondeson (1974).

similar to ordinary prisons, the "treatment" staff similar to prison staff, and the supposed patients were equally similar to the old prison clientele, only with an even more negative attitude towards what was happening to them than that which ordinary prisoners used to express. Indeterminate treatment for crime was obviously experienced as considerably more painful than old-fashioned intended pain.

Secondly: It was also shown that the system of treatment *did not successfully treat*. Treatment ideology was based on concepts of utilitarian and scientific thought. The protagonists of treatment made claims to be useful for the patient, and were at the same time open to research. But, as efficiently demonstrated in the literature on the effects of treatments for crime, the claims of usefulness have not been substantiated. Except for the death penalty, lifelong incarceration, and possibly castration, no cure has proved more efficient – as a means of preventing recidivism – than any other cure. Even in the few cases where there have been realities behind the terminology of treatment, no reduction in recidivism rates has been substantiated. The unanimity on this point just now is deafening, to an extent that makes it necessary to add some words of warning: what has been attempted has all the time been within the limits of available resources. Massive economic and social action has never been undertaken. Poor people have not been made rich, workers have not been given middle-class jobs, youth without anchorage has not been helped to realize hidden dreams, lonely people are not effectively given lasting new social relations. Of course they are not. That would demand social reorganizations far beyond the power of criminological research workers.

Thirdly, the concept of "dangerousness" was scrutinized. As von Hirsch (1972) summarizes in an excellent article, study after study had documented vague usage of the concept, low predictive ability when it comes to selecting the supposed dangerous ones, and the usual lack of treatment success. Scandinavian studies, Christiansen and others (1972), Dalgard (1966), and Stang (1966), fully agree. The endless row of scandals popping up around the few remaining special institutions (in autumn 1980 Reitgjerdet, in Norway, and Rampton in England) illustrate the impossible moral compromises built into them.

Science provided the arguments. But arguments are not sufficient to change social life. This brings us to a fourth point in the explanation of the defeat of the treatment ideology. In the 1960's, Labour had gained some power, or at least respectability. Spokesmen for the working class – but of course not necessarily coming from that class or belonging there except through ideology – were upset by the exposed inequalities and abuses disguised as treatment. It did not exactly strengthen the credibility of these measures that most receivers of this type of treatment for crime turned out to belong to just those classes supposed to be in political power. In addition came the fact that alternative measures of control seemed to be within sight. The concept of the welfare state had arrived. Poverty and misery ought to be handled by pensions and social assistance, rather than by prisons.

Chapter 4. Deterrence

4.1. The twin ideologies|

As one of those taking an active part in slaying the ideas and practice of treatment within the framework of penal law, I look with considerable anguish and anxiety on how deterrence is thriving on the death of its competitor. For a considerable period I have been lecturing on the fallacies of treatment during morning sessions in Oslo, while Johs. Andenæs[1] (1974) has argued for general prevention in the afternoon in the same room – to a very attentive audience. Of course they are attentive. These students are to man the system of crime control. They are in need of rational substitutes for the ideology of treatment. Good, rational, scientific substitutes – such as they are used to. They get them. And they get them in increasing numbers. During the last years we have received important proposals for a change in the penal system both in Finland (Straffrättskommitteens betänkande 1976) (Anttila 1977) and in Sweden (Brottsförebyggande Rådet 1977). Both declare the treatment ideology to be dead. And both find a most welcome substitute in deterrence – or "general prevention" as we call it in Scandinavia – as the basic foundation for the penal system. Dichotomies rule the world. Treatment-ideas have faded out, so there is a need for general prevention. To me this seems to be the major weakness in the otherwise inspiring and

---

[1] Johs. Andenæs is clearly the most important scholar in the development of ideas of general prevention. His first article on the topic is from 1950: Almenprevensjonen – illusjon eller realitet? (General Prevention – Illusion or Reality?) Most of his writings on the topic are published in English in the book *Punishment and Deterrence* (1974). For more critical Scandinavian views, see Aubert (1954) and Christie (1971).

inspired report on "New penal system" from Sweden (Brottsförebyggande Rådet 1977). As if treatment and deterrence were the only way of coping with conflicts.

It is too simple. But at the same time it is quite natural that ideas of general prevention are replacing ideas for treatment. The two sets of ideas are often presented as essentially different. But actually they are closely related on many points. They are both, in their recent stage, the outcome of an epoch of rational, useful thought. They have in common a manipulative element. Treatment is something intended to change the criminal; deterrence is an attempt to change other people's behaviour. It is in both cases pain with a purpose. In both cases some sort of behaviour-modification is supposed to take place.

Another common element is that they are both soundly embedded in science. But it is no longer any fun to measure the effects of treatment. They are all negative. Thus the researchers have moved to the new promised land. Is private killing deterred if state killing is introduced? Isaac Ehrlich (1975) claims 7 to 8 persons saved for each murderer executed, while other authors argue that Thorsten Sellin (1967) was right when he found that the death penalty was of no importance for the rate of murder in a state. The problems are more complex than with evaluation of the effect of treatment, but in principle the problems and potentialities for measurement are the same within general prevention and treatment. So also are the groups taking part in the new quarrels. Since there are questions of fact, of science and applied social engineering, we are again in the hands of measurement experts, as we shall later be in the hands of "social technicians" to get the results translated into action.

The similarities between treatment ideology and deterrence explain why they are so easily exchangeable. But there are also differences between the two. Particularly striking is the greater *survival ability* of the ideas within the field of deterrence or general prevention. The theory lays claim to empirical validity, just as treatment did. But it is a much more difficult topic to research. First, even its *basic concepts are vaguely delimited*. The unpreciseness within the area is amply illustrated by the simple fact that the key concepts "general prevention" and "deterrence" are used interchangeably throughout most of the literature, and therefore also here (cfr Andenæs 1974, Appendix 1). Furthermore, skimming the literature, one will see how everything from police activity to hanging can be classified as *stimuli* in a system of general prevention or deterrence. By and large, I think it is fair to say that everything that might be conceived of as elements in formal social control might also be characterized as elements in general prevention. And lastly: even in cases where the stimuli are pinned down to manageable proportions, the *effects* are often more troublesome to measure than when it comes to treatment. The reasons are again simple. Treatment effects at least had a formally clear target: those receiving treatment. With general prevention or deterrence these questions are more complicated. The general population, in whole or in part, is the target. That population might shift their activity from one type of crime to another, or move from one country to another, or might or might not have received the message of increased or decreased dosage of the stimuli.

Conceptually, as well as empirically, ideas of general prevention or deterrence are thus more cumbersome to handle than ideas of treatment. Looseness regarding definitions, stimuli, and target makes it next to impossible to disprove these ideas. The theory is strengthened by claims that it is founded on science, but survives empirical scrutiny. It is probably these aspects of the theory that make it possible for general prevention to fill the void after treatment has gone, and which makes the ideology suitable in an epoch where the infliction of pain would otherwise have been problematic.

4.2. Scientification of the obvious

It is obvious that punishment directs action. We know. We do not touch a red-hot oven. We do (often) change our behaviour if someone who means a lot to us blames us for misbehaving. More of us use seat-belts if it is expensive not to. What we know from our personal lives we tend to transfer to our public life. My experience in my family and circle of friends is given validity in the discussion on how to deter the thief, the drug addict, the violent offender. Why should not they become prevented by punishments, as I am by the hot oven?

There are actually rather good reasons why they are not. In the public arena there is no question of *immediate* control and punishment, but of formal sanctions following a long time after the possible crime. Here there is no question of punishments applied by one who has some relationship with the offender and therefore also greater possibilities than merely the creating of pain. Nor is it usually a question of punishments versus nothing, but of an increase versus a decrease of some sorts of punishments for specific types of crimes. To apply our daily experiences of pain avoidance to a general debate on deterrence, we would have to raise questions of the deterrence value of a red-hot oven of 200 C° versus one of 300 C°, or of a few minutes of scolding by a father against 15 minutes. And lastly and most important, a discussion of general prevention is not a discussion of the immediate effects of pain, but mostly of the effects on person A of the fact that person B is being punished. Some of us are not all that clever at learning from other people's experiences with their peculiar types of hot ovens.

Still, it is obvious that punishment does deter. Some sorts of punishment deter some actions in some situations. Without any punishments, chaos might emerge. When the police go on strike, trouble ensues. I agree completely. In its most elementary form, the basic premise of deterrence-theory is completely valid. If no action were taken against any of those who break the law, this would certainly affect the general level of crime in the country.

But that elementary form is not where ideas of general prevention or deterrence are applied in practice. In practice, these ideas are applied when politicians need arguments for increased penalties for certain crimes, or when judges want to be particularly harsh, e.g. increase a punishment from one to two years of imprisonment. Innumerable sentences in my country begin with the formula: "By reason of general prevention, it is here necessary to apply a severe sanction." It is a safe way out, one based both on intuition and on science.

And here we are at the core of the problem: theories on general prevention or deterrence are completely acceptable when it comes to the extreme examples, all or nothing. If no action were taken against those who break the law, this would certainly affect the general level of crime in the country. If tax-evasion were systematically met with capital punishment, it would likewise improve tax-behaviour. But these are not the cases where the ideas are used. Nearly all the concrete applications concern small additions or subtractions from usual standards of pain. Here theories and empirical studies within the field of general prevention give us no guidance. But by constantly using their extreme examples, the workers within the area give us an impression of having useful theories and results. They do in other words, give the process of pain delivery a false legitimacy. They could have said: We are of the opinion that criminals should suffer. This is a statement of values which is open to attack and we could have engaged in a moral debate on suffering. But they do not do that. They maintain, after complicated scientific discussions – and vivid demonstrations that ideas of treatment are without any scientific foundation –, that they base their own ideas on empirical science. And they produce all the classical cases of obvious effects of certain forms of pain to support their argument. By couching the obvious in scientific terms the impression is created that the choice of punishment is based on reason, and that the crime picture would have been different if the methods of punishment were different. Pain is given a scientific legitimization. We are not quite happy with what we are doing, but we persevere in the name of science!

4.3. Level of pain delivery

There are just now some 1 800 Norwegians in prison. This means approximately 44 per 100,000 of the population. But why just 44? Why not 115 per 100,000 as in Finland? Or why not take the large industrialized nations as a model? USA has half a million incarcerated just now, that means 230 per 100,000 of the population. USSR seems to have 1.7 million prisoners, that is 660 per 100,000 inhabitants, according to Neznansky (1979). But we could also make a complete turn-round and look at the case of a small, highly industrialized country with large minority problems, drug problems and crime problems, situated in the very heart of Europe: Holland with less than 20 prisoners per 100,000 of the population. That is in other words half the level of Norway, but exactly the same as Iceland, which for historical and geographical reasons ought to have resembled Norway. Internally in Eastern Europe we can find the same extreme variations with USSR and Poland at the top, while both Chechoslovakia and DDR seem to have very small numbers of prisoners.

Historically the picture shows even greater variations. At the time when Henrik Ibsen attempted to pass his high school exam – he failed – Norway had a prison population that was five times as high as in Denmark. Finland and Sweden had the same high figures. Our numbers of prison inmates subsequently fell dramatically until the turn of the century, since when – with the exception of Finland – they have kept at a fairly constant level, right up to the present day. They have kept constant, regardless of the fact that the figures in several crime indicators have doubled and re-doubled.

The point here is not to explain variations, or no-variations. The point is only to say that there is nothing new in an increase in the numbers of registered crimes without a corresponding increase in the number of prison inmates. Conversely, neither is it new for the level of registered cases to *go down* without a corresponding fall in the number of prisoners. There is no inevitable connection between the levels of crime and punishment. The two seem to exist in a complete and badly understood relationship to each other. There is little to indicate that the rate of crime in a country decides the rate of imprisonment. On the other hand, there is little to indicate that it is the rate of imprisonment, or the striking power of the police, which determines the level of crime. No doubt they do influence each other, but within a very wide area. For this and other reasons, to regard punishment simply as a means of control against undesirable activities is to adopt a far too restricted point of view.

4.4. Crime control as the goal for crime control?

Reading through the new wave of literature on deterrence, one is struck by the simplicity in the more basic reasons given for it all. It is the same simplicity that once pervaded the field of treatment. Then it was obvious that criminals had to be healed away from continuing their anti-social activities. Now it is equally obvious that the population, through examples of the sufferings of the sinners, have to be kept on the narrow track. It is as if the goal of the crime-control system is to control crime.

It cannot be. Or, let me restate it like this: if general prevention or deterrence had been the major goal of the operation, the crime-control system ought to have been constructed in quite a different way from what we find in our countries. If the goal of punishment was to create conformity, the crime-control system would have had to put hardly any effort into controlling those crimes which are perceived as serious crimes in our society. Most cases of murder might go unpunished; we know it is wrong, it would be more than sufficient to have some formal ceremony declaring who was to blame. Instead all the energy could be spent on the protection of weak norms. In Norway we have recently outlawed the selling of skate-boards. We have also passed a law making it compulsory to use seat-belts in the front seats of cars. Here are noble tasks for deterrence. Just a few five-year prison sentences, and we would have done it. Several hundred people would be spared severe bodily harm every year if the safety-belt law were obeyed; maybe thirty lives would be saved. That equals all the cases of murder in Norway in an average year.

It cannot be that simple.

A more sophisticated goal is suggested by Klaus Mäkelä (1975). He is one of the key persons behind the proposal for a new penal law for Finland, and his main argument is that the penal system, through general prevention, ought to create a priority list with regard to values in society. This is an interesting possibility. I shall soon come back to it. By and large, the idea has, however, been used simply to say that the more severe acts have to be met by the more severe punishments. Or, as stated in the major Swedish proposal quoted above: "The sanction ought to be dependent upon how dangerous or deplorable the crime is" (p. 200). So, most pain to those who have committed the most deplorable acts.

And who is to establish the priorities, that is, draw up the list? – Parliament is, in my part of the world. The pattern is simple: the penal law draws up the list of sins, Parliament categorizes and ranks them and decides in detail the amount of pain to be inflicted for each possible breaking of the law, and of course then allocates the greatest pain to the highest ranking sins.

With Klaus Mäkelä's formulation of a priority list with regard to values, the task has been broadened. The goal is not simply to control crime, but to give priorities to values reflected within penal law. This is also what the Swedish proposal for a "New Penal System" puts forward. It is not the need for control, but what the offence deserves which must determine the severity of the penalty – "The consequences must emphasise the danger or the atrocity of the crime" (p. 200).

But if this is the aim – and it can be a perfectly respectable aim – then new questions arise, in particular in relation to the understanding of what we actually are doing while talking like this. Is this really a discussion of general prevention? What are the scientific as well as social consequences of insisting that this is a discussion of general prevention? It is claimed that the murderer is executed not to prevent murder, but to denounce the evil character of murder. But why discuss this in the framework of an empirical analysis? Pain delivery is here used as a moral declaration. Why not say so?

By saying so, we would first of all weaken the position of general prevention. Furthermore, it would become even more obvious that pain delivery was intended to function as a sort of language. That would prepare the way for the idea that other, less painful languages, might be used. It would weaken the legitimization of inflicting pain when the pain was perceived as signals instead of concrete forms of controlling behaviour.

4.5. An opener to neo-classicism

Conceptually, as well as empirically, ideas of general prevention are more cumbersome to handle than ideas of treatment. But when it comes to standards of values, ideas of general prevention have considerable advantages. Ideologies of treatment were particularly efficient in blocking out questions of values. Based on an analogy from somatic medicine, treatment was seen as an obvious advantage. Treatment, and thus also treatment within the crime-control system, worked for the health of the client. Thus it was not appropriate to ask if the cure hurt. So many cures hurt. And it was not appropriate to ask if the client deserved the suffering; so much suffering is undeserved. And it was not necessary to control the healers, since there were no conflicting goals, only the honourable one upon which the client and society were agreed: to get the man socially healthy again – to cure him of crime.

Deterrence or general prevention is in quite a different position. Here it is clear that it is punishment we are talking about. It is intentional suffering. The penal system is there to hurt people, not to help or cure. And the pain is inflicted to further the interests of persons other than those brought to suffer. If those suffering are improved, it is O.K., but the principal target is the general public, as is particularly clearly stated in theories which use the term "general prevention". We are thus forced to see that interests are in conflict. We are forced to pay attention to the regulations of pain. With this description of the death of treatment ideology and the re-birth of deterrence, we have actually described two of the more important conditions for the emergence of what is now generally called the "neo-classical" movement. Let us turn to that phenomenon.

Chapter 5. Neo-classicism

5.1. Birth and re-birth

In order to describe the new classicism, it is expedient to take the old classicism as a starting point. A few words will suffice to give us some foundation. This classical trend was a true continuation of what is often known as the age of enlightenment. This age gave us Rousseau and Voltaire, and with it came a general underlining of the dignity and potentiality of man. (But with Rousseau, most definitely not of women.) In the field of criminal law, the movement was based on two main demands. Firstly, there was a demand for as little direction as possible over human conduct. Punishment should not exceed that which was necessary to prevent the criminal from doing the same thing again, and to prevent others from committing similar crimes. Secondly – and this was more strongly emphasized – there was a demand for a clear specification of what sort of sanction was to follow what sort of crime. Clarity and certainty became key words in the criminal courts. Both crime and punishment were to be clearly defined in advance. The punishment should be specified in detail according to the gravity of the crime.

It was the growth of the bourgeoisie in opposition to the aristocracy that lay at the root of this movement. The classical trend in criminal politics was sustained by the demand for protection from the oppressors' systematic arbitrarinesses. The bourgeoisie had grown in power and self-confidence to such a degree that it would no longer tolerate situations where a nobleman could get off with a fine whereas a commoner had to pay with his life. The demand was for equal punishment for nobleman and commoner in cases where the breach of law was the same. In order to secure this equality, the measure of punishment was to be firmly established in advance, according to the gravity of the deed, and not according to the social standing of the culprit or the discretion of the judge. The great scholars of criminal law, such as Beccaria and Blackstone, became great because they were great; but they also became great because their message was right for the times. It was compatible with the interests of a powerful group and with political and economic ideas and reasoning.

5.2. With Beccaria to USA.

Cesare Beccaria would nod with satisfaction if he were systematically to work his way through these three important books:

1. American Friend's Service Committee:
   Struggle for Justice. N.Y. 1971
2. Andrew von Hirsch:
   Doing Justice. Report of the Committee for the Study of Incarceration N.Y. 1976.
3. The Twentieth Century Fund Task Force on Criminal Sentencing:
   Fair and Certain Punishment. N.Y. 1976.

All three publications are a result of committee work. True, these committees were self-appointed, but they were all important, because of the integrity and calibre of their members, because of the position of these members in American society, and because of the strength of their arguments. In fact the titles of these books tell us a great deal. There is the *struggle* for justice, and then *doing* justice, and finally, when the term "justice" has been exhausted, we find the similar term "fair and certain punishment". Even then, characteristically, *punishment* – not treatment.

The first of these committees is an offshoot of the Quaker community in the United States. This fact in itself is important. It was precisely the Quaker movement which had introduced the ideas of corrective treatment to the USA, mainly on the lines of those in force in the Pennsylvania Prison, where the inmates were kept in complete isolation, each in his one-man cell, there to meditate upon their sins in undisturbed contact with God and the prison director, until they were fit to be discharged. As a reaction against this well-intended torture, later Quakers went in strongly for a completely time-fixed system under which punishment was meted out according to the gravity of the crime. Any other considerations not pertinent to the gravity of the crime would lead to an unfair allocation of punishment.

The second committee is usually called the von Hirsch Committee. It opened the way for certain exceptions from justice in the case of particularly dangerous criminals. It also allowed for an additional quota of extra time to be served by recidivists, and some reductions or increases in those cases where it was possible to produce evidence of mitigating or aggravating circumstances.

The third report can in many ways be seen as an operationalization of the second report; several of the members were also the same. Their system is, in their own description (p. 20), as follows:

For each subcategory of crime, we propose that the legislature, or a body it designates, adopt a presumptive sentence that should generally be imposed on typical first offenders who have committed the crime in the typical fashion.

The legislature also would determine how much the presumptive first-offender sentence ought to be increased for each succeeding conviction according to a formula based on a predetermined percentage. The theory behind this approach is that sentences for first offenders should be relatively low but that they should increase – rather sharply – with each succeeding conviction. Thus, we have suggested a geometric progression as the appropriate increment for more serious offenses: 50 percent "enhancement" for the second armed robbery, 100 percent for the third, 200 percent for the fourth, etc. The rise would, however, be less steep for petty offenders: 10 percent for the second-time pickpocket, 20 percent for the third, 30 percent for the fourth, etc.

The Task Force recommends that the legislature, or the body it designates, also define specific aggravating or mitigating factors, again based in frequently recurring characteristics of the crime and the criminal.

The concrete handling of mitigating and aggravating factors is described later (p. 46):

If the number of mitigating factors substantially exceeds the number of aggravating factors, the sentencing judge may reduce the presumptive sentence for the particular offender (presumptive sentence plus increment for prior convictions) by up to 50 percent. If the number of aggravating factors substantially exceeds the number of mitigating factors, the sentencing judge may increase the presumptive sentence for the particular offender by 50 percent.[1]

5.3. Beccaria in Scandinavia.

Publishers worked fast in the old days. Not more than 4 years after the original publication in Livorno of *Dei delitti e delle pene,* the book was translated into Swedish and published in Stockholm. The book was re-issued in Stockholm in 1977 in a beautiful Italian-Swedish edition. So, Beccaria would also have fared quite well if he had taken a study trip to northern Europe. Certain American details would have been missing, but in addition to the beautiful copy of his own book

---

[1] von Hirsch, followed by Judge Gilmore, dissents at this point and says that "The presumptive sentencing structure should also recognize that some mitigating or aggravating factors may be more important or serious than others and therefore could be assigned different weights" (p. 46). In the von Hirsch report, however, it is stated explicitly concerning aggravation or mitigation: "But such variations could not depart from the presumptive sentence by more than a prescribed amount. The limits on the permitted variations should be designed to preserve the basic ranking of penalties – and restrict overlaps in the severity of punishments for offenses of characteristically distinct seriousness" (p. 100).

he would have found much to please him, at least in two of four committee reports:

1. Straffrättskommitteens betänkande 1976:72. (På svensk: Band 1 og 2 1978) Finland. (Considerations of the Penal Law Committee 1976:72.)
2. Arbetsgruppen rörande kriminalpolitik. Nytt straffsystem. Brottsförebyggande rådet. 1977:7. Sweden. (Working Group on Criminal Policy. New Penal System. Advisory Committee for the Prevention of Crime. 1977:7.)
3. Stortingsmelding nr. 104 (1977–78) Om Kriminalpolitikken. Norway. (Parliamentary Report No. 104 (1977–78). Concerning Criminal Politics.)
4. Alternativer til frihedsstraf – et debatoplæg. Betænkning nr. 806. 1977. Denmark. (Alternatives to Imprisonment – A Debate Proposal. Report No. 806, 1977.)

Beccaria would have felt most at home in Finland, where it may be said that neo-classicism has had its strongest spokesmen. This is hardly mere coincidence. Classicism never quite lost its hold in Finland, which is natural in a society where the judicial system represents an important line of defence in foreign policy. In a Swedish summary of the Finnish edition of the Penal Law Committee's report, the conclusion is as follows:

To guarantee proportionality between crime and punishment, as well as the legal predictability, crimes within the new penal law have to be strongly differentiated according to severity so that the limits for punishment for each individual crime will be sufficiently narrowly delineated. To direct the opinions and attitudes with regard to law (rättsuppfatningarna) and the flow of information, one ought to mention typical punishments for each category of crime (p. 182).

In an article describing the proposals, a key member of the commission, Inkeri Anttila (1977, pp 103–104) states:

To make the system more clear there is proposed an ordering of all crimes in a limited number of severity grades . . . so that each category is related

41

to a fixed place on the scale of punishments. The very name of the crime should be sufficient to decide on the minimum and maximum punishments.

The Swedish proposals for a new penal system are more soft-spoken than the Finnish with regard to the demand for simple categories:

One must consider both the desire to obtain a clear and uniform practice in relation to the nature of the offence and the desire to be able to adjust the sanction according to the personality and social conditions so that future law-abidance might be accomplished (p. 405).

But this is immediately qualified:

According to the views of the working group, the gravity of the crime and the demand for proportionality between crime and punishment ought to be given a more dominant influence as regards the choice of punishment. Special rules must be created to do this. The necessary and natural reasons for such rules are well defined punishment scales in the catalogue of crimes, and specific rules concerning the internal severity of various means of punishment (p. 406).

That general prevention is the reason for punishment seems to be increasingly clear both in Finland and in Sweden. Inkeri Anttila (1977, p. 103) states:

The system has still, according to the committee, a major function in clarifying the content of and limits to the central prohibitions at the same time as it expresses the authoritative condemnation of disapproved acts. The punishment is first and foremost supposed to have a general preventive effect.

The Swedish report is completely built up around a discussion of the two alternatives: individual prevention (treatment) or general prevention. And at page 199 comes the conclusion: "We do thus recommend a penal system with a careful upgrading of the importance of general prevention."

The Norwegian report is very much like the other two in that it rejects the ideology of treatment for crime. What is different, and what Beccaria would dislike, is that the Norwegian report does *not* advocate any precise relationship between the gravity of the crime and the severity of punishment. Neither does it attempt to found the system on a basis of general prevention. Denmark has kept somewhat to the sidelines in the ideological debate, but has perhaps done more in practice through taking the lead in drastic reductions in the application of special measures based on treatment.

So far, so good. And I really do believe that what has happened is to the good – so far. The injustices within systems pretending to give treatment have been exposed by criticisms of such systems. The pains of punishment have been honestly exposed through the writings of the advocates of general prevention or deterrence. The need for protection against unjust pain delivery has been brought into focus by the neo-classicists. These have been necessary and important steps.

But now, when all that is done, what then is the next task?

My personal view would be: now the time is due, overdue, to stop any further advances of the ideology of general prevention, and also to prevent ideas of neo-classicism getting any further hold, at least within our Scandinavian societies. These ideologies have had a happy clarifying effect, they have triggered off necessary awareness. The simplicity and rigidity of neo-classicism makes it easy to see what it is all about. It also makes it easy to see that such a system is not acceptable as a foundation for a crime-control system.

Chapter 6. The hidden curriculum

Educationalists often talk about "the hidden curriculum". This is the message that is transmitted through the educational system without thought or design – indeed, without anyone necessarily being aware that it is being imparted. In schools the message may be that the most valuable, the most important knowledge in life is to be gained from books and, conversely, that those things which are self-taught are of less value. It can be that there is a correct solution, and only one solution, to most problems, and that this is to be found in text-books, or in the teacher. It can be the message that the basic way of learning is to gather into groups of equals, under the directorship of one, unequal, who knows the difference between right and wrong. It can be the belief that there are winners as well as losers in every system, often divided into standard groups according to directives from the authority. The winners will be rewarded, both in and out of school, whilst the losers lose everywhere. And it is the belief that the aim of scholarship is not learning for learning's sake, but to gain reward.

6.1. Crime is not important enough

The hidden message of neo-classicism lies first and foremost in the emphasis on the overwhelming significance of the criminal act. The violation of the law, this concrete action, is of such importance that it sets the whole machinery of the state in motion and decides in almost every detail everything that will subsequently take place. The crime – the sin –

becomes the decisive factor, not the wishes of the victim, not the individual characteristics of the culprit, not the particular circumstances of the local society. By excluding all these factors, the hidden message of neo-classicism becomes *a denial of the legitimacy of a whole series of alternatives which should be taken into consideration.*

Such a system becomes in fact a rejection of all those other values which should surely be included in this most important ritualistic display of state-power. Our criminal policies should reflect the totality of the basic values of the system. It is an affront to my values, and I think to many people's values, to construct a system where crimes are perceived as so important that they decide, in absolute priority to all other values, what ought to happen to the perpetrator of a particular crime. What does a neo-classical scale say about the value of kindness or of mercy? What about those offenders who have suffered so much beforehand in life that they, in a way, have been punished long before they committed the crime they now have to be punished for. What about the difference between the poor thief and the rich one, the brilliant and the stupid, the well-educated and the uneducated? I do not know. But I do know that I cannot accept a system for the ranking of values which by implication makes all these distinctions – and thereby the values they express – of negligible importance. A system that allows itself to be directed solely by the gravity of the act in no way contributes to a satisfactory set of standards for moral values in society. Neo-classicism solves some of the fundamental problems of priorities by simply ignoring them. It has thus an additional important, but again false, message: the world is simple, and all its sins can be squarely and clearly classified and ranked in advance.

6.2. Blaming individuals, not systems

The simplifications of neo-classicism do also lead attention towards individuals rather than towards social structures. Greenberg and Humphries (1980) clarify this in their analysis of the political consequences of the fixed sentencing reform (pp. 215–216):

. . . a just deserts philosophy focuses attention on the individual perpetrator alone. If I lose my job because the economy is in a state of contraction and then steal to support myself and my family – or if I am a juvenile and steal because the state has passed child labor legislation – or if I strike out in rage because the color of my skin subjects me to discrimination that reduces my opportunities – the just deserts model simply indicates that I should be punished for my wrongful act, though perhaps not as severely as I would be at present. One need not deny individual responsibility altogether in such cases to see that, in placing my culpability and the punishment I should receive at the center of attention, other topics are pushed to the periphery: the dynamics of the capitalist economy; the manner in which it allocates benefits and injuries among classes, races, and sexes – and in so doing generates the structural conditions to which members of the society respond when they violate the law; and the way class interests are represented in or excluded from the law. All these are neglected in favor of an abstract moral preoccupation with the conduct of the individual offender. But it is on precisely these excluded issues that a movement for radical political change must focus. The just deserts model interferes with this task, not merely by giving unduly abstract answers to the questions it asks (answers that neglect the social situation of the criminal actor), but even more by choosing to ask the questions it does.

6.3. Pain is not kind enough

Worse than the importance given to crime and individual blame is the legitimacy given to pain. Pain, intended to be pain, is elevated to being the legitimate answer to crime. But I learned in school, through the non-hidden curriculum, that the best answer was to turn the other cheek to him who struck me. Highly regarded solutions such as non-reaction, forgiveness and kindness are pushed into obscurity in the neo-classical simplicities. Neo-classicism attempts to create clarity and predictability. The system wants to keep the judge strictly controlled through specified laws, and thereby prevent arbitrariness. This makes it necessary also to specify the punishments. The detailed specifications represent an efficient protection for the criminal. But these specifications represent a heavy armour. The most doubtful aspect of the hidden curriculum reveals itself just here. Neo-classicism presents punishment as the inevitable solution, as a matter of course, by making it the only, invariable, alternative. Treatment ideology led to hidden punishment, secret infliction of pain, by pretending that cure or therapy was offered. But the new ideology punishes in the name of punishment. It makes punishment legitimate and unavoidable. I can well understand the old protagonists of treatment who exclaim with disgust: see what you have created, all of you destructive sociologists/criminologists in combination with human rights lawyers. Our ideas of treatment, they will admit, were often abused: they were often more words than realities. But ideas of treatment and their materialization *also reflected values*. Ideologies of treatment gave priority to many of those values you can now see fading away in the new classical rigid over-simplifications.[1] The reproof is justified. This does not mean that the pendulum should swing back to the old trend; but it does mean that the ideology of treatment, with its own vital, but often hidden, message of compassion, relief, care and goodness, should be taken seriously. The infliction of pain could be accepted in the

[1] I do fully agree with Stan Cohen (1977) when he states: "The much maligned humanitarianism which has been used to shield the otherwise unjustifiable positivist goal of 'treating' criminals, should not itself be obliterated. Once upon a time it was 'radical' to attack law, then it became 'radical' to attack psychiatry. As we now rush back to the bewildered embrace of lawyers who always thought we were against them, we should remind ourselves just what a tyranny the literal rule of law could turn out to be."

treatment ideology, but only as a link in a series of events which, in the long term, would improve the lot of the sufferer. That the pain inflicted was too great, and that it often took place with false aims, I need not enlarge upon here. But the ideology – and the acts – also contained realities of pain-reduction. Tony Bottoms (1980, p. 20) puts it this way: "The rehabilitative ethic, and perhaps still more the liberal reformism which preceded it, was an ethic of coercive caring, but at least there was caring".

Protagonists of treatment in countries that have never been through the stages of treatment ideology do often these days scold their Scandinavian colleagues for letting them down. They have attempted to humanize their penal systems by pointing to treatment in Scandinavia. In the meantime, the Scandinavians declare treatment dead, and thus make it completely impossible to modify old fashioned unkind penal systems.

In an attempt to counteract some of this damage let me just add: Treatment is out of fashion. But not all treatment. What has gone, at least in Scandinavia, is "treatment against crime", measures initiated to change the criminal tendencies of a particular person. It is the credibility of measures of control, most often disguised infliction of pain, that has vanished, but not the credibility of treatment or care of sick or suffering people. Prisons are filled with people in need of care and cure. Bad nerves, bad bodies, bad education – prisons are storing houses for deprived persons who stand in need of treatment and educational resources. Those fighting "treatment for crime" are of the opinion that humans should not be sentenced to imprisonment to give society the opportunity to treat them. But *if human beings are in prison to receive punishments,* they ought to get a maximum of treatment to improve their general conditions and soften their pain. Treatment for crime has lost its credibility. Treatment has not.

With the breakdown of the ideas of corrective treatment in criminal law, and the advance of neo-classicism, we have arrived at a most serious situation in our country, where the respectability of inflicting pain has been reinstated. We inflict pain that is intended to be pain, and we do so with a clear conscience.

6.4. Neutralization of guilt

Neo-classicism allows us to do this with a particularly good conscience. After all, it is not we, the power-holders, who bring these things about, but the lawbreaker himself. An automatic connection has been created between crime and punishment whereby, once the crime has been classified, the measure of suffering to be inflicted has also largely been decided. It absolves the individual executor from any kind of personal responsibility for the infliction of suffering. It is the criminal who first acted, he initiated the whole chain of events. The pain that follows is created by him, not by those handling the tools for creating such pain.

This whole tendency is strengthened by the overwhelming interest shown in neo-classical literature in the control of pain delivery, rather than in the pain itself. To regulate pain becomes more important – more in the centre of public and scholarly attention – than to use pain. Regulation of pain becomes so important that the necessity of inflicting pain is more or less taken for granted.

Regulation is given so much attention that little attention is left for discussing the qualities of the regulated commodity and whether this commodity actually is all that necessary. This becomes a new way to create distance to pain. Sufferings disappear in a fog of regulatory mechanisms. Somewhere, far behind, is an activity of dubious repute. But we do not come quite close to it because we are so intensely preoccupied with building up regulatory mechanisms.

6.5. The strong state

The neo-classicists also have a hidden message when it comes to the image they present of the state. Their system presupposes the existence of a strong state, and they strengthen that state even further. Their system is very far from one where the parties feel their way through constantly changing solutions adapted to the needs of the present situation. Their questions are not of the type: Is this really an act that ought to be labelled crime . . . what would be the consequences of perceiving it as stupidity, youthful horseplay, or maybe exceptional heroism . . . are no solutions other than punishment possible . . . what about compensation, or maybe some cooperative activity? With neo-classicism it is all a question of pre-established laws, equally binding for all human beings in all situations. As a safeguard against arbitrary decisions, by state or despot, the laws must be firm. But it seems evident that this safeguard at the same time constitutes a barrier to alternative solutions.

The Scandinavian advocates for the recent blend of neo-classicism and general prevention are quite clear on this point. They might differ considerably in their views on the relative merits of capitalism or Marxism, but they have interesting similarities in their views on the state. Johs. Andenæs gives us a glimpse of his conception in his most recent article on general prevention. He says: "If one looks at law-making and crime control as one large piece of machinery with the task to direct the behaviour of the citizens, then . . ." Klaus Mäkelä (1975) concludes with a statement that the purpose of the penal law is not limited to the prevention of crime. Its purpose is in addition to "reproduce the official morals and thereby itself" (p. 277). Inkeri Anttila (1977) states that the penal law committee emphasized that the penal law system could not be the only or even the major means for directing the citizens' behaviour in accordance with the goals of official policy *(samhälls-politikens målsättningar)*. But the system has still, according to the committee, a basic function of clarifying the content of the central prohibitions and their limits while at the same time expressing the authoritative denunciation by society of disapproved acts.

At first sight the situation appears different in the USA. The psychoanalyst Willard Gaylin and the historian David Rothman have a joint and very emotional introduction to the von Hirsch report (1976):

If progressive reformers shared a basic trust in the state, more eager to involve its power in the society than to limit it, we as a group shared a basic mistrust of the power of the state. At the least we suspected that discretion might cloak discrimination and arbitrariness. We were certainly not prepared, a priori, to construct a system in which the benevolent motives of the administrators were sufficient reasons to cloak them with power. (p. XXXII).

But when we go into the report, and Gaylin and Rothman were both members, quite a different picture emerges. Here it is described how that power, taken away from the administrators, is to be used in their combined system of classicism and deterrence. For example, when it comes to the question of the level of punishments:

The difficulty is the absence of data: the deterrent impact of an untried scale of penalties is not known. It will be necessary to choose the scale's magnitude on the basis of surmise – on a best guess of what its deterrent effect is likely to be. Once a scale has been implemented, with its magnitude chosen in somewhat arbitrary fashion, it can then be altered with experience. If the magnitude selected leads to a substantial rise in overall crime rates, an upward adjustment can be made (within the upper bounds of commensurate deserts). If no such rise results, it would then be appropriate to experiment with further reductions diminishing the scale's magnitude in stages and observing whether any significant loss of deterrent effect occurs. (pp. 135–136).

A system is created where the whims of the administrators are exchanged for an enormously powerful, simple and centralized system of state control. Neo-classicism, as expressed in the spectrum from Ervin Goffman in the von Hirsch committee to Police Chief Joseph D. Mcamara in the Twentieth Century Fund Task Force, has created a system that both needs and strengthens a strong centralized state.[2] Their Scandinavian parallels are in the same situation.

The defeat of treatment ideology for crime and its practice was a necessary first step. It cleared the ground and brought some severe abuses of power against the weak to an end. The neo-classical school, with its rigid system for demanding a year for an eye and three months for a tooth, was probably both unavoidable and on balance a good second step, at least until such a system became law. The simplicity and rigidity in neo-classicism makes it relatively easy to see what it is all about. When guilt, recidivism, and aggravating as well as mitigating circumstances have been quantified, the remainder is simple arithmetic. But when we do see it all, and particularly when we see it in a system that claims to be there to establish a ranking order of values, then I must admit that I am very far from being happy. That society is not, by choice, my society. It is a centralized, authoritarian state which, in the eagerness to create equality, has to block all those softer values from being considered at all. As an alternative to this we must create arrangements to enable us to cope with the task of re-establishing a situation in accordance with the total value pattern within the social system.

---

[2] It all seems to be a replication of the Becker/Gouldner debate from the late sixties. That debate started with an important presidential article by Howard Becker (1967) on "Whose side are we on?" Becker declared himself clearly on the side of the underdog, fighting prison officers, guards, administrators and bureaucrats. Al Gouldner's (1968) caustic comments were that the unintended consequences of the defeat of the middle men would be more power at the top.

Chapter 7. The computer

The treatment ideology emphasizes the character of the individual offender when choosing the line of sanction. The neo-classicists place the main emphasis on the character of the crime. Both extreme positions of the pendulum lead to the loss of advantages offered by the opposite position. In this situation, it is tempting to try to combine the two approaches, to get the best from both of them. With a little help from computers, that might be accomplished.

Computers have an unlimited capacity. They could create order. They could combine all relevant individual attributes and give an accurate prediction of possible recidivism. At the same time they could take into consideration all important characteristics of the criminal act and of the relevant mitigating or accentuating circumstances. The importance of every factor could be given a predetermined weight. Lombroso and Beccaria might be equally satisfied. This is not Utopia. This is the system that has been worked out by Gottfredson, Wilkins and Hoffman (1978) for the federal Parole Boards in the United States in connection with decisions on parole for prisoners who have been given indeterminate sentences. The system is in full use.

The system has several great advantages. It has enormous capacity. It can include as many factors as we want. It is reliable. Equal factors carry equal weight in all decisions. When correctly instructed, the computer will always give equal cases equal treatment, quite independently of the number of factors taken into consideration. The system might also be characterized as the most democratic, in the sense that it is the legislators and not the administration who decide the moment of discharge. Wilkins can ask the legislators or the central deciding body to determine exactly what relative weight should be attached to every conceivable factor to be considered, such as type of crime, extent of injury to the victim, bedwetting as a child, level of education, risk of recidivism, or conduct in prison. The law may, for example, impose two months' additional sentence for each year of education beyond the normal level (the prisoner should have known better!) or, if desired, two months' remission for each year of higher education (the more highly educated suffer more from punishment). The system also offers the best possibility for *administrative control*. One can read off in a minute the increase of prison inmates it would lead to if serious drug crimes were upgraded by x points. The system of the calculating machine is also closely related to the ideas of *general prevention*. It can preach its gospel not only to judges, but to the entire population. In a few years most industrialized nations will be able to receive details of flight and train timetables, restaurant menus and prices direct on the television screen. We will be able to press the buttons and get the answer in a moment. It will be even simpler, since fairly stable charges will be involved, to connect up standard penalties for every type of crime carried out under every kind of circumstances by every conceivable type of perpetrator. This will be a truly rational form of prevention. Ask your own home-computer and you will get the exact answer to the question what a contemplated breach of the law will cost.

But there are also problems.

First and foremost, the computer is perfect, infallible. When it is correctly programmed, its decisions are obvious. After guilt was decided, nobody would need to attend before the judge to listen to his decisions if they themselves had some mini-computers at their disposal. This means that *chance* is taken away from court-decisions. In civil cases, this would lead to a situation where nobody used the courts. The outcome would be known; why take the trouble?

If ideals demand that the courts should be used, a certain degree of uncertainty – not complete uncertainty, just enough to make it worth while trying – seems to be necessary.

Another possibility would be to make an attempt to change the computer-programme. This would be the major strategy in criminal cases where – granted that he was found guilty, and most are – the mini-computer might tell the criminal that the outcome would be highly undesirable. Here a second limitation created by perfection dawns upon us. It has to do with the question of *who* should have the right to decide on what is put into the computer, and also how much it should count, that is what sort of weight should be given to it.

Here we can think of a vast number of alternatives in the decision-making bodies. Decisions could be made by:

The United Nations in the General Assembly

The United Nations in the Crime Committee

Regional bodies such as the European Council or the Union for the Arabic States

National Parliaments

State Parliaments – such as the Californian legislature

Sub-units of politicians – such as the Parole Boards or Law Committees within the legislature

A random sample of the population questioned through the telephone or personal interviews

A sample from the county, or county representatives

A sample from the municipality of the victim or the offender

A totality of those close to the victim or the offender

Or the decisions could be made by the victim and the offender in cooperation.

This list is, as you will see, organized so that the decisions on the content of the computers – the norms that will decide the outcome – are brought in increasing proximity to those concerned as we go down the list. You will also observe that the moment the proximity is perfect, then the computer is also completely superfluous. In that case, people can talk, directly. It is in the United Nations end of the scale that computers are unavoidable. In other words, whether or not the computer is a good and necessary thing within penal law depends on the character of the decision-making system. At the same time it is clear that the very existence of the computers represents a temptation and probably also a pressure towards giving higher priority towards those types of decision-making systems that can make efficient use of computers. Those who dislike such systems will be negatively inclined towards the use of computers within this area.

This leads to a third, and maybe the major, problem with computers within penal law. It is not only the parties that do not need to go to court, since their mini-computers could tell them the outcome in advance. But the judge does not need them there either in cases where guilt is clearly established. Why should he? Every category to be considered for sentencing is strictly defined in advance. If he is given the necessary information that makes it possible for him to fill in the correct number in the category, he has no need to see the criminal. Since the categories are agreed on as relevant, and are known in advance, the judge could simplify his task by asking the parties to deliver written information on the relevant points and order his secretary to clear up any possible disagreements on relevant information before he started the process of sentencing, that is, before he touched the button on the computer for the final answer.

The computer in penal law has through these elements double ability to create distance. Decisions on relevance – the computer rules – can be made very far away from the parties concerned. And when they are applied, the parties need not be there. Decisions on pain can thus be made in complete insulation from those who are to receive sentence.

Here will be no distraction caused by sorrow and tears, by sweat and swear. It will be more like a bureaucracy. Documents, clean desks and – better than in any bureaucracy – clear answers. It will be those answers needed to allow society to remain stable. The principles in the answer will have been decided by people far above. The concrete answer will be exactly similar to the answer given to all criminals belonging to the same category. And the answer is clearly initiated by the criminal himself. The judge has no other responsibility than to push the button.

A fourth point with computers has to do with their hidden curriculum. Their hidden message is that conflicts are there to be solved. Computers are calculating machines, they are designed to give answers. But is it so obvious that answers are what is called for? Is it the final outcome that is of primary importance in criminal proceedings, or is it the process? I will come back to this in the next Chapter.

Training in law is training in simplification. It is a trained incapacity to look at all values in a situation, and instead to select only the legally relevant ones, that is, those defined by the high priests within the system to be the relevant ones. Neo-classicism is just a logical extension of that whole process of elimination. So few elements of the totality are considered that complete equality is guaranteed. But it is, through its simplifications, a primitive system. Computers open the way to new, complex possibilities. But now when a technical tool for perfection has been created, we are able to see more clearly that complete clarity, predictability, and pre-programmed behaviour suited for administrative control can never be the only ideals for any legal system. Neo-classicism is maybe an oversimplified attempt to reach a goal that never was. Maybe law is closer related to art than most of us are aware of. But art and power do often stand in a strained relationship.

Chapter 8. Neo-positivism

8.1. The impotent society

After the meetings of the International Sociological Association in Sweden in 1978, I received several letters from colleagues abroad asking for explanations of what they had seen. The meetings took place in Uppsala, only a short journey from the capital, Stockholm. They had been there, and they were shocked and bewildered by what they had seen: the drunks, the drugged, young derelicts roaming about, gathering at the doorsteps of Parliament, the major concert hall, in the subways, dark spots on an otherwise immaculately clean, beautiful, Scandinavian design. Police were in attendance, but very seldom interfered. Several participants had also travelled through the other Scandinavian countries, and had been struck by the same thing everywhere. In Oslo, one of the favourite hang-outs for small traders and users of drugs is a hillock in the park at the doorstep of the Royal Palace, with the Old University and the National Theatre as the closest neighbours, and Parliament just in front. It is as if these young drop-outs want to be seen, as if they want to say something.

Maybe they do.

There are several interpretations of what they are saying. The simplest is that they are not saying anything at all. At least not anything new. They have always been around and have now only become more visible. It is just a question of old figures against a new ground. We have torn down the worst slums. The natural meeting-points for the *lumpenproletariat* have been eliminated, converted into pleasant, dull, clean blocks for dull, clean, adapted families. In the absence of ghettos for the losers, they gather around the centres of pride. If Harlem and its equivalents did not exist, they would gather outside the Rockefeller Center.

Another interpretation concentrates on the position of youth in modern, industrialized societies. Youth has become a highly prolonged stage of life. The age structure has been adapted to the work structure. People are less needed for work than before. We take care of this by increasing the number of years spent waiting for work, and pensioned off after work. The general age for retirement is gradually being decreased. We call it a privilege, and so it is for many. At the other end of the age scale, we increase the number of years people are kept outside the work force by increasing the number of compulsory or close to compulsory years spent in the educational system. That system is open to everybody. It has been the pride of our social democratic countries. Everybody is given the privilege to compete – on an arena built by and for the middle classes. It is an arrangement perfectly suited for transforming structural in-equalities into experience of individual failure and guilt (cfr Hernes and Knudsen 1976, Callewaert and Nilsson 1978). Most losers are good losers. They accept the verdict, they are not better than their grades, and they do also accept the position in or outside of the work force deserved by the grade. But some do not. They sit it out in the park.

Ivan Illich (1978) has made a case for the fruitfully occu-pied unemployed. In Denmark, a group of unemployed have created a society for enjoying their happy free status. Free-dom from the slavery in the types of work given to large groups of the working population is a great privilege, for those given the resources to enjoy it. But it takes a long life and lots of training in classical languages and upper class puritanism to create one of those idle Englishmen who enjoyed life on inherited means. It took a Jesuit training and considerable natural talent to create an Illich. Useful unemployment is beyond the reach of most people in societies where we are programmed to follow the rhythm of days and years of work. The unemployed or pensioned are literally paid off, given free time without content. They will easily end up in life-styles beyond their own and other peoples' control.

In addition comes the factor that class-differences are more visible now. Seen from abroad or from the perspective of old people, and measured in money or material belongings, most people are unbelievably wealthy within our Scandinavian societies. But people do not look at themselves from abroad or in a historical perspective. Inequalities remain, and the *growth* in wealth which could temporarily soften dissatisfaction has come to a stop. Inequalities are not any more only a preliminary stage. They are seen by all parties concerned as permanent features of societies with explicit emphasis on equality.

If these societies are of the Scandinavian type, they will designate themselves as welfare states. Hasse Zetterberg has called these societies a gambler's paradise, a place where you can only win, not lose. It was in the sixties he coined the term in a lecture in Oslo. I am not so sure he would use it today. It is possible to lose completely, drug addicts prove it every day. Prostitutes exemplify it. The minimum pension for old or sick people is in Norway close to one fourth of the average salary of an industrial worker. Those dependent on money from the municipal social security system might end up with less than half of the minimum pension. As formulated by Knut Dahl Jacobsen (1967), "the greatest hindrance towards attaining the welfare state is the belief that we have one." Balvig (1980) has made a strong case showing that the old relationship between poverty and crime is still in existence, regardless of all talk to the contrary.

Nonetheless; we live in some sort of welfare state. Those

belonging to the conforming poor cannot lose *completely*. For them there is a safety-net somewhere far below. This is the big difference from the beginning of this century. Our old labour politicians look with a deserved pride on their accomplishments. These are societies where the "deserving poor" are not starving, have some sort of shelter, and are also given some sort of material care during the very last stages of life.

But this very system creates certain peculiar problems for social control. Parts of the *lumpenproletariat* have lost close to everything. There is nothing more to take away as punishment. They cannot be controlled by a threat of losing work, they are out of it. They cannot be controlled by any threat of losing family-relations, they have none. They cannot be controlled by the threat that relatives will suffer; the welfare state is supposed to take care of them. The belief that we have one is as useful for members at the bottom as for those more privileged when it comes to calming guilt for lack of attendance to relatives or friends in need of care. And lastly; those members of the *lumpenproletariat* willing to live at the absolute minimum cannot be starved into control. They will be assured the basic minimum even though they are often forced to convert it into drugs or alcohol.

The time is free, the miminum-money is mine (and could not be removed without shaking the whole base of our welfare societies), and nobody needs me anyhow. Why should I not drink or drug myself to any stage I want. Any stage, including my own death.

In addition comes the recent history of crime control as described in this book. Treatment for crime seems to be of no use. Science, as well as social developments, have killed it all. Compulsive treatment of deviant behaviour did not work, and it was clearly demonstrated that the idea of treatment resulted in severe injustices directed against members of the working class. Treatment institutions for young offenders, dangerous offenders, and psychopaths are nearly all abolished. Forensic psychiatrists have got a very low status among doctors. The younger generation has up to now nearly all been against all sorts of compulsory treatment for most types of deviant behaviour. As a reaction to abuses in the name of treatment, and to forestall potential abuses in deterrence theory, we have got a more legalistic ideology, exemplified through neo-classicism.

We can still cope with severe crime, that is, we can get the severe offenders off the streets in the name of justice. But when it comes to the small ones, we are impotent. They are easily seen. It is a disgusting sight. They drink or dope themselves to death. But some do it on a pension, others on petty crimes difficult to prove. Treatment would not help.

8.2. Advocates for control

Not only visitors from abroad have difficulties in comprehending the highly visible phenomena of dark deviance on the otherwise so clean and well-ordered surface. We all have difficulties, but some more than others. Three groups are particularly heavily hurt:

First: Parents and others related to youngsters who drop out with drugs, alcohol, or general criminal activities. Those who did not obey parental authority could be starved back into the herd in the olden days. Nowadays they can survive on leftovers from affluence plus social security. Vocal requests for alternative measures of control are therefore increasingly being made. We cannot let young people run completely wild. Compulsory attendance in schools, treatment-homes, collectivities and eventually prisons becomes the declared alternative to work. Some old liberals are attempting to stem the tide by pointing to the dangers of stigma and the horrors of prisons. They are easily neutralized by parents pointing to a child lost in drug abuse. They would rather see him alive, in prison. I agree.

A second vocal category consists of the actual or potential victims of visible crime. It is impossible to say whether crime has increased or not. But it seems to be certain that anxiety concerning crime has increased. Crime is such an important part of the commodities sold through the mass-media. At the same time, the social structure has changed in a way that makes it impossible to find out how representative these news reports are. Balvig (1979) has clearly documented that the anxiety for being a victim of crime increases the more isolated a person is. The lonely old lady will see the same as the foreign visitor in the centre of Stockholm. In addition, she will read the newspaper and get it all confirmed. But she is not the only one. And there are realities behind the concern. The welfare states have had a considerable success in distributing property. There are few grown-ups without belongings, things that can be stolen, property for which they demand protection through stern measures against intruders.

Again some old liberals attempt to intervene, telling the old ladies that it is not all that dangerous, and pointing out to the new, affluent worker that those who threaten his property are sad, bad cases, poor and sick, and in need of understanding rather than pain. The former Minister of Justice from the Labour party in Norway said so, but she became former through such sayings. The political far left seems confused and in doubt as to how to handle this matter at present. Most take a liberal position, but there are exceptions, as represented by the influential Maoist Jan Myrdal (1977). In several articles he has argued that criminals are the enemies of the working class. Police and prison guards are according to Myrdal closer to the working class than the *lumpenproletariat*. It is according to him far from obvious that the worker in all cases ought to support demands from the prison movements. "We are in favour of law and order. We are at the side of the police both in the fight against crime, and in the policemen's fight for improved working-conditions and increased salaries".

It was back in the 1960's that prisoners and former prisoners held their first general meeting in Sweden. The press called it "The thieves' parliament". It came as a shock. Prisoners should keep quiet, not make demands, not interfere in the penal process. A few years later, all the Scandinavian countries had their prisoner organizations. They were in the centre of public attention. They worked for the improvement of prison conditions, they organized prisoners, they organized strikes. Thomas Mathiesen (1974) describes it well. They experienced many defeats, but also some victories. The most important effect of it all was probably an increased feeling of self-confidence and dignity among the participants of the movements.

Today, the situation has changed dramatically. These days activities within the prison movements tend to be much more defensive of positions attained in the beginning of the 1970's. The movements are not any longer in the centre of public attention. The climate has changed. Former allies have become enemies, more soft-spoken, or out of power. An economic recession makes for less willingness to experiment. The highly visible dark spot on the welfare facade strengthens those forces demanding action, not softness. Demands for law and order have also had a breakthrough in Scandinavia. Of course they have. Highly industrialized societies are bound to create situations where that will happen. During the first stages, when there was always more of everything, more to distribute, we could all relax, liberalism could rule, problems could be defined as transitory. Now they are permanent. There is not more to distribute every year. The situation has changed from one with a perceived potentiality of unlimited progress, to one of defence of what has been attained.

But more embittered, and also more confused than any,

are the architects of it all, those who were young and poor and active in a fight for a socialism later converted into a social democratism, later converted into a welfare state. Compared to our past poverty, our recent affluence is beyond imagination. Studies (e.g. Ramsöy 1977) show it, and we do not even need the studies, since so many still remember. Compared to past insecurities, our recent social security system has outstanding qualities. Is it not obvious that we have reached the goal, that we are there? Why do they then remain, those thin, pale youngsters outside the Palace, visible both to the King and all the King's men?

The temptation must be tremendous. Just a few decisions in Parliament, and the last dark spot would be removed. It would not be necessary to call it a law against hooliganism; that might be misunderstood. One could call it a law for the protection of problem-youth. They need protection. Their parents need it. Their victims need it. The welfare states need it now that they have come so close to perfection that they lose control.

To sum it all up: The situation is one where minor offenders have become more visible and also more difficult to control at the very same time as their relatives, victims of crime, left-wing politicians and architects of the welfare states have become vocal advocates for some sort of action. In its totality, this is an unstable situation. Something is bound to happen, and so it does.

8.3. Our comrades

Last summer, 350 social workers met in Sweden to receive the message on how to handle the drug problem. They met in a small and geographically very remote place called Hassela. Nothing is more known, more debated in social work circles just now than Hassela. Institutions based on their principles are mushrooming, also in other Scandinavian countries. And their ideas are also invading other types of institutions as well as ordinary social work practice.

And what is the message?

The most pronounced theme is that the clients are our comrades. The drug-users and drinkers, they belong to the working class. We, the Hassela-people are socialists. They are our comrades, and must be treated as such. We have a common identity and a common cause. Comradeship means responsibility. we are obliged to drag our comrades out of their misery by any means available. Any. From 1850 and up to the turn of the century the Scandinavian workers suffered through their enormous alcohol consumption. The leaders of the labour movement saw this, and acted. Workers could not become free, and the movement strong, if alcohol was not controlled. Teetotalism became an important part of labour, and the alcohol problem was brought under control. Now consumption of alcohol as well as drugs is back to the old, dangerous level, and has to be controlled by the old recipe.

One of the old ways was to *force* people into abstinence. Comrades are not allowed to drug themselves to death, they are rescued. You die for your comrade and of course you compel him to live. If necessary, you compel him to stop using drugs. If necessary, you enforce your comradely attention for several years, until he is rescued. Hassela is for young drug users. They are picked up in Stockholm, sent to Hassela independently of their own wishes and brought back by the police if they run away. They are kept one year. In addition comes one year of compulsive attendance at a "folk high school" together with other youngsters whose stay is not compulsory. They can be kept until the age of 20. The legal base for keeping them is the Child Welfare Law.

Another major theme is the general moralism of the

approach. Standards are established, breach of standards severely censured by staff-members and other comrades. Hassela is not a place for digging into clients' souls, nor into the many sad external circumstances in earlier life. There is no soft liberalism here. This is a demanding place with heavy consequences for a possible lack of response or lack of responsibility. It is a rough life. Rough for the youngsters, but also for the staff. They live there, take part in all activities, have no shield between themselves and the others. It is a total institution for all.

It seems to work. They claim success rates far above anything experienced in the Kingdom of Sweden these days. This is a controversial matter (Englund 1975, Thelander 1979), but the claim might prove to be substantiated. Hassela is probably very successful in bringing young people's drug use to an end, and has most certainly proved successful in reducing the feeling of acute professional impotence among social workers and related professionals. The costs of that success might outweigh the gains of their help to young drug users.

8.4. My comrade, the functionary

The problem with Hassela is not Hassela, but all those eagerly waiting for a message on what to do in all those situations where society today does not act at all. Hassela seems to be filled with warm idealism and with people who live with the consequences of their ideas. I have great respect for their acts. But not for their social analysis. The analogy between our Scandinavian societies in this century and the century before is an extremely dangerous one, omitting the existence of the category of people most eagerly receiving their message. During the last twenty years we have had an enormous expansion in the number of professionals trained into an identity of caring for other people's behavioural problems. Now they are there, some of them with their identity at stake. But at the same time they are functionaries, most of them working in bureaucracies, from nine to four, with clear lines of command, with documents, with short encounters with clients, with potential power vis-à-vis these clients, but just administrative power. They will not have to live with the consequences of their decisions; they will drive home to the suburbs, to partner and children and dogs and summer-house, and somewhere someone will have to let drug-users feel the consequences when they do not live according to the rules of a game between comrades. Those someones will become the new breed within social control in westernized societies. I suggest we call them comrade-functionaries.

But some will do more than talk as comrades but act as mere functionaries. They will start collectivities for drug-users themselves. They have learned how to do it. If clients run away, they will try to find them and bring them back. If they cannot find them, they will ask the police to do so. When the police bring them back, they will keep a close eye on them, and prevent them from running away anew. But they will get tired. Partners will need attention; their children have got the measles; the police get irritated; they install some locks. But locks are easily opened, and illegal opening is a challenge in itself. A fence is raised, some clients dig a hole; a wall is raised, some jump the wall; bars are installed, some remove the bars and jump the wall. A special treatment unit is built.

It is like an old film. We have been through it all before. The potentialities of the Hassela ideology reflect a repetition of work schools for criminal youngsters. They started as idealistically run and completely open offers to young people who really deserved an honest offer. Through the mechanics of teachers being obliged to keep their unusually unwilling pupils, they ended as unusually unpleasant indeterminate prisons. It is difficult to understand why social workers should prove more successful.

The special arrangements and institutions for children difficult to govern were established in Scandinavia at the end of the last century as a result of combined interests among law personnel, educationalists and politicians (Stang Dahl 1978). It came as a great relief to everybody on the controlling side. The staff should be experts, to a large extent recruited from education, health or welfare. But this last element never materialized. There were not so many professionals around in those days. But now there are, eagerly waiting for new tasks, and also protected against the memories from past approaches by seeing themselves as comrades. We end up in a system of enforced consumption where one of the commodities becomes social control, served by a comrade-functionary close to that type of personnel we otherwise meet in totalitarian societies.

Chapter 9. Pain forever?

9.1. A one-dimensional pendulum

Like heavy waves, the various forms of crime control appear, disappear – and appear again. Or maybe a picture of a pendulum in motion would be better. A pendulum with classicism and positivism at the extreme positions, later exchanged with neo-classicism and neo-positivism. None of the extreme positions are stable. They have a built-in potentiality for change. The classical and neo-classical positions take care of equality according to the gravity of the act, but not of a more broad concept of justice. Nor are these positions able to create a machinery for control of the minor types of crime or deviance. The positivistic and neo-positivistic positions give an excellent base for control, particularly of minor deviance, but also of the extreme forms such as the habitual or the dangerous criminal. Their defects become visible in periods when the need for such a type of control is not so strongly felt, or where the potential targets for this type of control gain in political strength or support.

Is there then no calm ocean, no peaceful position or middle stage where the pendulum stops moving, where harmony is established? Probably not in theory, but certainly in practice, established through blurred compromises. A bit of each. Some equality based on the gravity of the offence, some control of minor offenders based on their supposed personal needs, some indeterminate sentences based on a hypothesis of dangerousness. Crime control is not based on clear principles. Not any more than vice control or control of the international economy. It is a day-to-day matter, workable through compromises, protected by unclarities. Few social systems would survive if the participants understood each other completely, or were fully governed by the declared basic principles of their system.

One reason why compromises are so easily reached within the crime-control system might be that the extreme positions on the pendulum are not that different after all. Maybe the *similarities* between positivism and classicism, as well as between neo-positivism and neo-classicism are greater than their differences.

I have earlier argued that treatment ideology and general prevention (or deterrence) have basic similarities. Now I want to push the level of provocation one step further, and argue that positivism and classicism – as they appear within the field of crime control – also envisage some fundamental similarities. Beccaria punished with a purpose. The von Hirsch report establishes the level of pain delivery so as to be able to prevent crime. They fought for equality in pain delivery. But the delivery had a cause. Behind it all is the obvious goal of crime control. Neo-classicism is not only activated by the revival of interests in general prevention. The two are in a harmonious relationship. Just deserts would be only an empty shell if it were not seen as a regulatory mechanism for pain with a purpose.

Pendulum moves between classicism and positivism represent a true picture when the task is to describe the major practical important positions in the debate on crime control. But it is an untrue picture if the intention were to give an analysis of fundamentally different positions within the area. The pendulum I have described up to this point is in a way a one-dimensional one. There is another dimension, by and large ignored by makers of criminal policy and neglected – or mostly frowned upon – by sociologists as well as liberals. Let me try to bring us a bit closer to this alternative position. But it is a difficult task, so let me hasten slowly.

9.2. Experts needed

A murder has occurred. It is in a normal-sized modern town of let us say, 300,000 inhabitants. You read about it in the newspaper, and get very upset. Two evenings before you had listened to a lecture given by the supposed killer. You did not notice anything unusual about the speech, nor about the speaker. The whole affair becomes incomprehensible. The judiciary also seems to find it incomprehensible. They declare that psychiatrists will be called upon, to explain.

But let us imagine another killing. This time 200 years back in time. To ensure that some of us have some common stock of knowledge of the scene of the murder, we can this time imagine that it happened in Hilltown in New England, that decaying town made famous through the penetrating description by George Caspar Homans (1951). If we had lived in Hilltown at that time, we would probably have found it ridiculous to call in an expert of the mind to explain why the killer had killed. Ridiculous because we all knew why he killed. Maybe not in advance, and not so certainly that we would have dared to interfere to prevent the murder. But after the act, we would not have been surprised, and we would have agreed between friends that this was exactly what we all could have expected all along.

The difference between the experience of the two killings has to do with the amount and type of information the participants would have about each other. So many people live in a middle-sized modern town that it is impossible to know them all. In addition, life is organized in ways that only allow us to have segmented knowledge of other beings. We know fellow-workers as workers, friends as friends, family members as family members, . . . We have a narrow basis for predicting behaviour outside the exact group we meet. In Hilltown, pretty well everything was known about everyone.

The challenge to the psychiatrist is in many ways to recreate the lost Hilltown. The good psychiatrist will recreate the totality of the killer; he or she will dissolve the boundaries around the segments of the killer's existence and thereby make it possible to grasp the incomprehensible. By doing this, the psychiatrist will do the same job at the level of the individual as the sociologist attempts at the social level. We have become foreign to each other (and thereby also often to ourselves). We need experts to pull us together. The same has happened to societies. We need help to re-create the totality.

There are reasons for the developments of the various branches of experts. Good, scientific reasons. We need the experts, just as we need most of the other providers of service in modern society. We need the doctors, the nurses, the hospitals, the schools. But they also need us. This brings me to the other side of the coin. Experts need clients, and might create them in the process. This will often make us forget that we are not quite so foreign to each other as some writers make us believe. Some do still live in the countryside. And some never do leave their neighbourhood within their Megalopolis.

9.3. Subterranean patterns

Let me include a story from our valleys. It sounds like a fairy-tale, but it is true enough, observed and written down by a perceptive student (Bjørkan, 1977). Her task was to find out about the ancient but still highly active Norwegian institution of *"lensmann"*, that is a sort of sheriff, but with numerous civil tasks in addition. He lives in the district. Very often the position was passed on from father to son. In old times, he was often a bad character, in alliance with the rich and the mighty. Therefore, in the folk-tales, he was the one to be outwitted, while the King was more kind, and stupid.

Today the *lensmann* is more under control, more common, more popular, and dependent on his popularity to be able to function. He directs auctions, sees to it that unmarried mothers get their money from runaway fathers, – and controls crime. And here comes Bjørkan's major point. When interviewing the *lensmenn,* she found they all reported that there was no crime in their districts. A few exceptions occurred. People passing by might sometimes break into a petrol-station or shop. But the people of the valley? Never.

But as already mentioned, Bjørkan was a perceptive observer, and while she was conducting the interview, several episodes occurred. The telephone rang, a lady had lost her purse; the *lensmann* asked his assistant to drive down to the close-by cafe, the purse was found and brought back to the lady. So was the young man who was using the purse. He happened to be the lady's son.

Another episode: A report came in on breaking and entering into a store of weapons for the home guard. The *lensmann* jumped into his car, drove far up into the mountains in the direction of the store, met a car high up there, stopped the car, found Ole drunk as usual, with a carload of guns to irritate his father. He brought Ole home and took the guns to a more safe depot. What a cliff-hanger story lost for the mass-media! Helicopters and anti-terrorist police might have been engaged in the crime-hunt of the century. Now it was only Ole. An old story of misery and family quarrels.

Crime is not a "thing". Crime is a concept applicable in certain social situations where it is possible and in the interests of one or several parties to apply it. We can create crime by creating systems that ask for the word. We can extinguish crime by creating the opposite types of systems.

9.4. Counter cultures

Denmark is a society for collectivities. Not only collectivities run by functionaries, but also real ones, run by ordinary people. What machines divide, man can draw together. Christiania is the largest one. It is situated in a beautiful area, close to the heart of Copenhagen, formerly used by the army, abandoned, and then occupied by slum-stormers evicted from housing close by, and later joined by others. The number of inhabitants is unknown; those living there have no great affinity with systems of registration or public statistics, but they are more than a thousand, spread out in some large stone buildings and a considerable number of small wooden ones. The material standard of living is generally extremely low. It is possible to survive there on very little money. Some inhabitants work in Copenhagen, outside the collectivity. Several receive social benefits in one form or another. Inside Christiania there are also some possibilities of making a living. Several work-shops have come into being, restaurants, a bakery, a health-centre based on "natural medicine". One of the most interesting theatres of Denmark has its home base in Christiania. In a way the whole place is like a huge, burlesque performance.

It is a terrifying place; dirty, untidy, "hash" is sold openly, a lot of drunks, and an overwhelming number of strange-looking people, some obviously insane, nearly all as if taken out of a medieval painting. Lots of children, partly living with their parents in Christiania, partly run away from Denmark to the Free Town of Christiania, establishing a group called "Children's power". A great number of dogs, remarkably nice dogs, run all over the place; several horses are kept there. Once in a lonely part of the area, I met a brown bear. It did not feel right – according to Christiania values – when I slowly realized that the bear was chained.

The place has its ups and downs. My last experience was

in the Grey Hall. Two thousand people were crammed in to initiate a fight against the use of hard drugs in Christiania and in Denmark. In the following period, very strong pressure was exerted on sellers and users. A national movement was created, and Christiania moved upwards. But it is a society with great scepticism against leadership, any leadership. Observed from a distance, it looks as if natural leaders are born, again and again, when crises emerge. Taking responsibility, they become visible both inside and outside Christiania. But thereby they break with the rule of equality, and lose their potentiality to act. The same has been observed within the feminist movement. So, Christiania cannot be ruled. But it cannot easily be killed off either. Each time an attempt is made, it mobilizes enormously, and the government hesitates.

Christiania has many friends. As Berl Kutchinsky (1981) puts it so well: liberalism is important in Denmark. And Christiania itself is an important part of Denmark. In addition to the dirt and sin and misery, it is also an expression of core values of Danish society. In the good periods – but remember there are also bad ones – this is a place for communal living. Since so many work so little, they have more time than usual for talk, cultural activities, and mutual attendance. At the same time, however, there are clear indicators (Madsen 1979) that commercialism is important inside Christiania.

Christiania is a challenge to Denmark, but maybe the more ordinary Denmark will in the end take over from the inside.

Christiania is a sort of medieval town, based on a mixture of small private enterprises and communal sharing. At the other end of Denmark is another collectivity, one based more on hard work and socialism. Its name is the "Tvind-schools", its symbol the largest windmill in Denmark, built by the participants. It has grown out of the folk-high-school movement of Denmark, a strong current of that country, mostly with Christian affiliations, a place of development and learning for youth after they have gone through the compulsory school. The teachers at Tvind put all their salaries into one hat and share. It is a very efficient technique applied by a minority within a capitalistic welfare state. The Tvind-system has become rich, and buys more and more farms, which they convert into schools.

An essential element is that the pupils as well as the teachers work and study at the same time. They have built their own buildings, invented their own sewage system, now copied in several places, and their own electric power system. The windmill gives a surplus of electricity, sold to the electricity companies. If you do not know how to repair a broken window or carburettor, you just have to try. Of course you can do it. They buy old buses, convert them into class-rooms, and drive all over Europe and Asia to study the living conditions and to become able to report home in lectures and speeches from real life, not only from books. When abroad, they attempt to take part in ordinary peoples' life, often through some joint projects in villages or cities. In addition to the "Travelling folk-high-school" they operate a teachers' high school, and a so-called "After-school" for young people just out of the compulsory school system. Work is a core value. The discipline is very strict. Alcohol and "hash" are absolutely banned, even in vacations. Breaking these rules means eviction.

Christiania and Tvind, they are both a part of the surrounding society, but also in contrast to it. And they stand in contrast to each other. The abundance of time in Christiania, the shortage of it in Tvind; the lack of discipline in Christiania, the abundance of it in Tvind. The danger of Christiania seems to be too little intervention, tolerance to an extent that might endanger life. The danger of Tvind is a collective attitude so strong that individuals might become crushed. But still, what unites the two systems is something more important. It is basic trust in human beings. Christiania and Tvind are societies of anti-clients. Through their concrete practice, they declare that humans can accomplish what they really want to accomplish. Man is a creator, not a mere consumer.

This spring, thirty persons held a meeting on the West Coast of Norway. They gathered to discuss ethical and philosophical questions, as well as very practical ones, such as how to organize their daily life and get the necessary work done. They kept on for three days. Except for a few invited speakers, they were all, according to our official system of classification, mentally defective.

Were they?

This is an uninteresting question. They had their meeting. Their discussions were interesting. After the meeting, they all went home to four different villages where they have their permanent life. They all work. They all take part in decision-making. They are all engaged in various cultural activities. There is a totality in the existence which gives it qualities beyond the usual.

They are supposed to be dumb. I was thinking of that the other day during an evening meal in one of the villages. We were probably ten people around the table. Two or three had no "official handicap", others had several. Vidar asked if we wanted more tea, and served us all, quietly, no mess, not a drop was spilt. In addition to being designated mentally deficient, Vidar is blind. But the point of the story is not that the blind, classified as mentally deficient, Vidar, served tea. The point is the behaviour of the remaining persons around the table. It was a matter of course that Vidar should serve us tea. It was an atmosphere of confidence. I think I observed a slightly watchful glance on the face of one who had taken particular responsibility in setting the table; but no interference, no comments afterwards. This was no result of planning. I asked an old aquaintance the next day. No strategy, it had never been discussed in the household.

The only threat I can envisage against the circle of people around that table, is that there might be too many helpers around. Not professionals, they are banned from this community, at least in their capacity as professionals. But do-gooders. It is a very realistic threat. Young people are enormously attracted to this community. They queue up to take part. Too many would easily mean that they would take the teapot away from Vidar and maybe even push him out of his major job in the household: drying the dishes. He does it, once a day, in addition to his other job outside the household. To protect Vidar and others, dishwashers are not allowed into the system. Also to protect him, some of the young people who would otherwise be tempted to give too much help are forced to take their meals in a ghetto where there are none of the formerly declared mentally deficients, no insane, no blind, no crippled. In other words the situation has been turned exactly upside down. The youngsters have become the handicapped, those to protect the others against. And the young people know it. They strive to get access, to get close to a totality, to get teachers of all sorts, that is, from the whole variety of mankind, in vital questions. This is not only a counter-culture as Teodore Roszak (1969) would have called it. It is a counter-society, more radical than any I know of, more so than Tvind and Christiania, more than any political movement. In the midst of our well-regulated, immensely affluent societies of providers of service, even here there are counter-forces, societies of anti-clients, places where it is not obvious who are the providers and who are the receivers.

Vidaråsen is the name of the collectivity Vidar lives in. (The similarity in names is probably a coincidence.) Officially, Vidaråsen is an institution for mentally handicapped persons. It receives money from the State. As in Tvind, all salaries are put in a hat and shared. Collectivities of this type were first created in Scotland by the German refugee Karl König. His inspirer was Rudolf Steiner. Internationally, they are known as Camphill villages. They show interesting similarities to the French type of villages called "Larche", created by Jean Vanier (Clarke, 1974). The ground seems particularly fertile for such villages in Norway. There are four of them, with plans for two more to come. Just now, they are striving to get the authorities to redefine them from being institutions for handicapped people into being communes for such people who for one reason or another find life in large, compartmentalized units unsuitable. Vidaråsen could not function without subsidies from the State. It is a reaction against domineering features of the welfare state. At the same time it is a form of life dependent on that state, yet possessing potentialities for the renewal of the welfare state.

Of course they are belivers, as we all are. In Vidaråsen and Camphill they have the same idea with regard to souls as are found in so many belief-systems. They think that the soul, when a body dies, passes to another body. This is a hypothesis with great consequences for social life. It makes people very attentive. External signs such as blurred talk, eruptive bodily moves, or permanently running noses do not become all that important as indicators of who you are. Inside might live a dignified soul. When we look hard, they are proved right.

Chapter 10. Some conditions for a low level of pain infliction

With these indeed all too short sketches as a common stock of information, we might be able to discuss some possible conditions for a low level of pain infliction. Let me organize that discussion around five basic categories: Knowledge, Power, Vulnerability, Mutual dependence and Belief system.

10.1. Knowledge

The importance of knowledge might be best illustrated in the contrasting features of a society of experts versus the subterranean pattern suggested through the stories from our valleys. All other things being equal, but obviously they are not, it seems to be a plausible hypothesis that the greater the amount of information on the totality of the life of the relevant system members, the less useful (and needed) are generalized concepts such as "sickness", "madness", – and "crime". The system members come to know so much about each other, that the broad concepts in a way become too simple. They do not add information, they do not explain.

In Norwegian we have the word "*bygdeoriginal*". "The odd local character" might serve as a translation. Small-scale societies are not characterized by similarity in ways of presenting oneself, or in general behaviour. On the contrary, they exhibit a most colourful variation in the gallery of persons. A large amount of our older literature is filled with descriptions of them. These are not flat societies where everybody is and behaves just like everybody else. But such societies are often characterized by continuity in the highly individualized life styles. *"Bygdeoriginalene"* are persons created through a long period of interaction during which the parties get sufficient time to get to know each other. In this type of society, we find a great amount of variation *between* persons, but not so much *in* the person. Eccentricity is tolerated, but inconsistency is not. It becomes a tolerance of variation in the sense of consistent differences from the usual ways of behaving. It becomes tolerance of patterned behaviour so closely related to a specific individual that it might be called a personality trait. Strange people are tolerated, but their roles are not for hire.

But with so much information regarding the system members that the simple generalized abstractions do not suffice, the most simplified reactions towards unwanted behaviour do not suffice either. Crime *and* punishment. The two concepts are at the same level of abstraction. In a social system where the one is not useful, the other might not be useful either. Knowing the *"bygdeoriginal"* – the odd local character – the system members will understand his behaviour to an extent that makes one aware of the complexities in changing it. Simplified punishments will not be seen as natural and obligatory answers.

It is important to realize that not all small-scale societies have knowledge about their members. Smallness is no guarantee of knowledge, while at the same time some large systems contain considerable mutual information between the system members. A very important factor here is the question of how long the system has been in existence. Small societies *without a common history* will have no place for individualized deviance. There has not been the time, nor the encounters necessary, to create such roles. In a small-scale society with a limited amount of mutual knowledge between the system members, the demands will often be great for *similarity in behaviour*. Non-conforming will be categorized in abstract terms, and censured by simplistic actions. Systems with limited internal interaction will remain without a common history. Modern "dormitory towns" are exemplary cases. The extreme cases should probably not be called systems at all, since so little interaction is going on. Not even punishments will create interaction, since external police are called in and the rest of the procedure of punishment is done outside the system. To arrange the situation in a way that forced those who lived there in the non-system to cope with a breach of conformity without possibilities for exportation of the problem, would in itself help to create a system of the non-system. The need for pain infliction might thus be reduced through system-creating.

Another essential factor limiting common knowledge is segmentation. A small caste society might keep the participants efficiently separated. The effect of this will of course be increased through inequalities in power.

10.2. Power

People with power can deliver pain. Power means the ability to get other people to do what you want them to do, independently of their own wishes. The penal judge is above the defendant. He is protected by the symbols of the courtroom, the elevated bench, the robe, in some systems also the wig, the prestige of the building, the atmosphere, his training, affiliations, special class, and enjoys the advantage that the decisions are in reality made somewhere else; the judge is only carrying out a heavy task. His heart is bleeding, but he is obliged to act, to punish.

People without power are in quite a different situation. If they have no protection, or they are not strong, pain delivery is not a tempting alternative. The potential receiver would not take it. He would hit back. Intentional infliction of pain is easier the further away the recipient is from the deliveryman. Milgram (1965) has shown it experimentally. He hired people – in the name of science – to give electric shocks to other people. The hired ones were brought to believe that the object of the study was to find out whether people would learn faster if they were punished for mistakes. Few were hesitant to apply punishment, even when they thought the voltage was dangerously high. But they became hesitant the closer the victim was brought to them. I have similar data from a study of behaviour in concentration camps (Christie 1972). The more prisoners were able to define themselves as ordinary human beings vis-à-vis the guards, the closer they came, the greater were their chances of survival. These prisoners were Jugoslavians in Nacht- und Nebel-camps in the North of Norway. Those who were able to learn the essentials of the language were protected, at least against intentional extermination. They made their guards vulnerable to the guards' usual standards of behaviour against usual humans. By talking, the prisoners became individualized and humanized. They came so close that punishment was seen to be what it really was.

Here we are at the heart of the matter. We saw how the neo-classical approach objectified the process of punishment. The choice was in a way made by other authorities, and by the criminal who started the whole thing. The judge became only a tool, an instrument of destiny. Delivery of pain is converted to the appropriate scientific method, and the yardstick is the gravity of the crime. The whims and wishes of the judge are of no importance, nor are those of the criminal. With a little help from computers, they do not need to meet at all. In other words, the whole situation is unusually well designed for a process of pain-inflicting.

If there is a conflict, and some people are given the task of doing something about it, we are faced with two alternatives. One is to give those people power. If so, that power must be controlled. Neo-classicism is one way of controlling power. Elaborate possibilities for appeal from the decisions of the power-holders is a related one. So also are training, professionalization and all sorts of "objectifying mechanisms" such as rules of competence, protection by rank, and selection by qualifications. The solution at the other extreme is that those given the task of handling the conflict are not given power. The dwarf at the royal court symbolizes the idea; so small that he was unusually well suited as a go-between – until he became a specialist, and was therefore regarded as potentially dangerous. The child might sometimes take on this role in a family conflict. Or one whose advanced age made him an outsider might take the role. The other symbol on this side is the independent third party – asked to help, but not given authority to enforce, and with no possibility of personal gain related to the outcome of the conflict.

10.3. Vulnerability

A way of controlling power is to make the wielders of power vulnerable. Vulnerability might be established in several ways. Three are particularly important. They are vulnerability through equality in status, through equality in qualifications, and through close and available physical proximity.

The importance of proximity is exemplified in the recent discussion of neighbourhood-police. As a reaction against the alienated conditions in many urban areas, several attempts have been made to decentralize police services as well as social and health services. It is again an expression of one of the many pendulum moves in society. After having destroyed municipal police systems, the numerous small police stations, the small health units, and the general practitioners in so many areas of life, it is now in vogue to re-create them. Police cars and electronics did not quite make up for the loss of that old constable Bollingmo who patrolled my neighbourhood in my early childhood. So, we re-invent him. We do, as in Oslo quite recently, convert some caravans into local police stations, allocate a permanent squad to serve there, and make serious attempts to let the police come closer to those they ought to serve. It is at the same time an attempt to become able to control the controllers. Police cannot be controlled through bureaucratic means. As Stökken (1974) has underlined, police work leaves little trace on paper, if the police so wish. That makes control from above close to impossible. The alternative is control from below, from the public in contact with the police. But to make that type of control efficient, the police must be converted into a neighbourhood-police.

There are, however, sceptics around. Stan Cohen (1979) and Thomas Mathiesen (1978) are among them. The core of the critique centres on Focault's (1975) concept of the disciplined society. And they are right. These become uneven relationships. Prisons might be abolished by a method that makes the whole society into something similar to it. Within the police, it is not old constable Bollingmo we re-create. It is a stream-lined officer integrated in quite another way into a huge, army-like unit with great striking capacity. The electronics are there, and the cars. The new "local" policemen are only local in the sense of being there while on duty. They have no lasting commitment; they leave the beat after service-hours. They leave for a life unknown to those who remain. In other words, they are not vulnerable. The old local policeman was. He had of course his status as a policeman, and he could call for assistance. In bad cases he could mobilize the power of the State. But he would not call in external authorities all the time. He was in so many ways a hostage of his community. He lived there, or close by. His children were in their schools, his wife in their stores. This was not a case of the iron fist and the velvet glove (Cooper 1974). This was a case of real vulnerability.

In contrast to this, a decentralized system of control by personnel anchored outside the system might easily convert into a system of espionage completely uncontrolled by the system-members themselves. To avoid a perversion, the idea of a decentralized police service presupposes a police force dependent on the neighbourhood it is to police, with weak links to the police force outside the neighbourhood and with important changes in the organization of the ordinary police. If we let the neighbourhood police expand, we must shrink the central police and block the communication channels between centre and periphery. The police must be seen as a total system. If we just *add* neighbourhood police, we come dangerously close to "the punitive city" so well described by Cohen (1979). The vulnerability of the police has to be preserved.

"Special qualifications" represent another shield against vulnerability. Experts on social matters have that form of defence. They are certified as more competent than others on social matters. They are trained in a language peculiar to their equals. They will come to the local office for social matters to serve the community, but will easily end up as rulers. More than the policemen, they are out of control, seen from the locals' point of view. They are not designed to let people cope with their conflicts, but to solve the conflicts for them. And as judges, they are preprogrammed to disregard certain possibilities, and put emphasis on others. But in contrast to judges, they are not trained into a realization that they are handling conflicts. They will, like the old treatment personnel within crime control, easily convert into pain-delivering persons under the disguise of being health personnel.

With increased insights regarding the dangers of power and the needs for vulnerability maybe the time was ripe to re-establish the respectability of the Child Welfare Boards and the Temperance Boards we have in most of Scandinavia.

Again a pendulum move; after heavy criticism of the boards, now back to the boards! But it would have to be back to a different type of boards than those operating today. It would actually be a form much closer to the law-makers' original intentions with these boards, only with some changes due to our experience up to now, and because they are to function in a different society. These new boards would not be the domain of the child savers (Platt 1969). We have gained experience. We will man them with equals. Nor would they get power. We know more now about the paralysing effects of power on social systems. Respectable boards would not get functionaries either. They would consist of members, not rulers. And lastly, but important for the boards' possibilities for useful functioning, they would operate in a completely new social setting. The old boards came into being in societies where poverty was still an important fact of life. The child savers from the last century are probably less open to criticism when evaluated according to their own time. Ours is the post-welfare state in the sense that the supply of basic social needs is to a large extent taken for granted.

10.4. Mutual dependence

Social systems do not waste essential members. Verner Goldschmidt (1954) was instrumental after the second world war in writing down the first "non-penal" criminal law of Greenland (or Kaladlit Nunat – "the land of the human being" as that continent is called after the establishment of some independence from Denmark). The law represents an attempt to codify Eskimo traditions and views. And a strong theme in Goldschmidt's writing is the emphasis on peace-making and limitations on loss of system members. To create a situation where a good hunter loses face means a risk that the local community loses the man. The community would therefore resort to other means.

Emile Durkheim (1933) differentiates between societies based on organic versus mechanical solidarity. He finds organic solidarity in societies with a highly developed division of labour. Here participants become dependent on each other; they exchange services, and thereby become mutually controlled. The contrast is a society of equals, where the members are in a way glued together through similarity. Durkheim calls it a society based on mechanical solidarity. With modernization, societies move, according to Durkheim, from mechanical solidarity towards organic solidarity, and punitiveness decreases.

I can follow Durkheim all along, with the exception of the last sentence above. Durkheim was indeed a product of the French urban culture. He quotes with approval a statement that if one has seen one Indian, one has seen them all, while it is obvious that among civilized people two individuals can immediately be seen as different. This bias has probably made him blind to the amount of variation in small-scale societies, and also to the problems of control within the large ones. Since he believes that small "primitive" societies consist of equal persons, he sees limited reasons for exchange of services. But then he is losing what could have been his best example of organic solidarity: a small-scale society with lots of mutual dependence *and where the participants cannot be replaced*. Here organic solidarity can be said to function at its maximum, and so does also the parties' possibility of exercising mutual control. In large units, conditions for solidarity are more limited, since role-incumbents might so easily be exchanged. We can buy them at the labour market and use the leftovers as targets for pain.

10.5. Belief system

The collectivities described in Chapter 9 allow us to approach this problem. Tvind does, to a certain extent, apply punishments, even though eviction is its major form. But Tvind is a highly centralized system with inequalities in authority and a great circulation of members who do not come to know each other that well. Christiania cannot punish because there is no one in authority. Vidaråsen cannot, because the idea is impossible.

That is no explanation, I know, so let me try again. Let us move back to the supper-table. Let us think that Vidar drops the teapot, intentionally. I cannot think he ever would, but let us nevertheless try to think of it.

First, to inflict pain on Vidar – what might that accomplish? To Vidar, who is so kind, so complex, who has problems enough, whose total biography many know and whose total existence just now is known to everybody around the table: delivery would not just be delivery, and the pain would be everybody's pain. There is too much shared knowledge in the system.

On the other hand: In a system like Vidaråsen, power is not equally shared. It cannot be denied that some people are in many ways quicker than other people. They are thereby able to get their way, and they are protected against counter-sanctions. This is obvious, but compensated by a belief-system. Vidaråsen has one which keeps power under control, which makes people equal. If the body is only a shelter for a dignified soul, the system members are brought into positions of mutual respect. They become respected equals to an extent that makes pain-infliction a rather far-fetched idea. In addition, they have ideas that it is more right to serve other people than to use them as servants. This again restricts the possibilities of using other people's suffering as a means for the upkeep of law and order.

But of course, this opening for the importance of beliefs is also an opening for the importance of beliefs that *ask for* pain. The Palace of Inquistions at Cartagena is such a beautiful building. Here they lived in dignity and comfort the kind priests, with the chamber of torture just one floor below. And I use the word kind without any irony. I am convinced that many among them were just kind believers in God, rescuing the poor souls. To the inquisitors, Hell was a reality, and they delivered pain with a preventive purpose.

Chapter 11. Participatory justice

11.1. Civilization of conflicts

Once upon a time, most roads for innovation within the field of criminal policy were one-way roads. It was more or less taken for granted that ideas first appeared in the most industrially developed countries, and then gradually spread to the less highly industrialized ones. Experts from Europe or the United States of America travelled to Africa or to Asiatic countries to convey the message; reports on Scandinavian prisons were export articles. This still goes on, but with some marked changes. Some of the representatives from some of the highly industrialized countries are no longer all that sure that they have a message, or at any rate the whole message. It is in this situation that the roads for ideas have changed over to two-way traffic. If anything is clear, it is that several of the less industrialized countries have to a large extent applied *civil* law where we apply criminal law. Especially in societies that lack a strong central power, where the State is a weak one, or where the State representatives are far away, people are forced not to apply force.

What do they do instead?

First, it is important not to presuppose that conflict *ought to be solved*. The quest for solution is a puritan, ethnocentric conception. For most of my life I have taken it for granted that the outcome ought to be a solution, until I was kindly made aware of my limited perspective. Then for a while I clung to an alternative concept: "conflict management". Again a narrow, ethnocentrically determined choice. To manage, the word is related to the Italian expression to train a horse for the manège, or in our time, managers, the word for those who direct other people. It is very far from a participatory term. Conflicts might be solved, but they might also be lived with. "Conflict-handling" is probably a better term. "Conflict participation" might be the best. That term does not direct attention to the outcome, but to the act. Maybe participation is more important than solutions.

Conflicts are not necessarily a "bad thing". They can also be seen as something of value, a commmodity not to be wasted. Conflicts are not in abundance in a modern society; they are a scarcity. They are in danger of being lost, or often stolen. The victim in a criminal case is a sort of double loser in our society. First vis-à-vis the offender, secondly vis-à-vis the state. He is excluded from any participation in his own conflict. His conflict is stolen by the state, a theft which in particular is carried out by professionals. I have applied this perspective in an article "Conflicts as property" (Christie 1977), and will therefore not go into further details here, except for one quotation, which tries to illustrate the most important loss when conflicts are stolen (p.8.):

This loss is first and foremost a loss in *opportunities for norm-clarification*. It is a loss of pedagogical possibilities. It is a loss of opportunities for a continuous discussion of what represents the law of the land. How wrong was the thief, how right was the victim? Lawyers are, as we say, trained into agreement on what is relevant in a case. But that means a trained incapacity in letting the parties decide what *they* think is relevant. It means that it is difficult to stage what we might call a political debate in the court. When the victim is small and the offender big in size or power – how blameworthy then is the crime? And what about the opposite case, the small thief and the big house-owner? If the offender is well educated, ought he then to suffer more, or maybe less, for his sins? Or if he is black, or if he is young, or if the other party is an insurance company, or if his wife has just left him, or if his factory will break down if he has to go to jail, or if his daughter will lose her fiancé, or if he was drunk, or if he was sad, or if he was mad? There is no end to it. And maybe there ought to be none. Maybe Barotse law as described by Max Gluckman (1967) is a better instrument for norm-clarification, allowing the conflicting parties to bring in the whole chain of old complaints and arguments each time.

Again we are close to a most important difference between the neo-classical approach in penal law, and a general aspect of participatory justice. In penal law, values are clarified through a gradation of the inflicting of pain. The state establishes its scale, the rank-order of values, through variation in the number of blows administered to the criminal, or through the number of months or years taken away from him. Pain is used as communication, as a language. In participatory justice, the same result – the clarification of values – is accomplished in the process itself. Attention is moved from the end-result to the process.

11.2. Compensatory justice

But civil law is of course not just participation and words. Acts are supposed to follow. If things are wrong, they must be righted. Peace must be reinstituted. Particularly the victim must be compensated. In all systems without a strong state, victim compensation seems to be the major solution. It is what social anthropologists to a large extent report on. It is what legal historians describe. And it is the system we apply ourselves when we have hurt other people and feel, or are brought to accept, that we have to put things right.

Victim compensation is such an obvious solution and used by most people in the world in most situations. Why is it not used at the state level in highly industrialized countries? Or at least, why do we not immediately, with added insight, extend the system of victim compensation, and let the domain of penal law diminish? Three reasons often given are close to the obvious. Let us look at them in turn.

First it cannot be done in societies of our type. Ours are societies of specialization. We need experts to handle crime.

I will soon go into this problem in greater detail. Here it suffices to mention that not all social arrangements are there because they are necessary. They might also be in existence because it once was a good thing for those with power that they should come into existence. Later, the arrangement continues by the very fact that it also serves other interests. The servants of the courts are well served by themselves. So are also their auxilliary personnel.

Secondly; Compensatory justice presupposes that compensation can be given. The offender must be able to give something back. But criminals are most often poor people. They have nothing to give. The answers to this are many. It is correct that our prisons are by and large filled with poor people. We let the poor pay with the only commodity that is close to being equally distributed in society: time. Time is taken away to create pain. But time could be used for compensatory purposes if we so wished. It is an organizational problem, not an impossibility. Furthermore, it is not quite true that prisoners are *that* poor. Lots of young apprehended criminals have the usual range of youth-gadgets; bikes, stereo-equipment, etc. But the law and those running it are surprisingly hesitant to take any action to transfer any of these belongings from the youngsters to the use or benefit of the victim. Property rights are better protected than rights to freedom. It is simpler to take away a youngster's time than his bike. Property rights are important to us all. Imprisonment is highly improbable for the ordinary citizen. In addition, those medieval sinners who were dealt with through systems of civil justice were not always all that rich. Herman Bianchi has in an article (1979), and also in lectures, described how sanctuaries functioned in those days. Churches and monasteries functioned as places where offenders could not be touched. Thus they became bases for discussions between representatives of the offenders and victims about guilt and compensation. A killer might be forgiven if he promised to pay 1000 guilders. He was then free to leave the monastery. But it might later become clear that he was not able to pay the 1000 guilders. In this case he was also a bad man, but less so. He was now converted from a killer to a debtor. New discussions might follow, and the parties might agree to reduce the debt to a size that could realistically be paid. A little to the victim was better than the life of the criminal to the state. Offenders completely unwilling to compensate were slowly and subtly pushed down in rank and comfort within the sanctuaries, and eventually out of them as refugees to other countries, or as crusaders in the combined fight for Christianity and trade privileges. Herman Bianchi is now engaged in attempts to re-establish sanctuaries in Amsterdam. That is one of the few original ideas within our field in the latter part of this century.

But here comes the third objection: this would lead to the most terrible abuses. The strong victim would squeeze the poor offender out of all proportion, or the strong offender would just laugh at the victim if compensation were mentioned. Or vendettas would threaten. Victims and their relatives or friends would take the law into their own hands, and the offender and his gang would do the same. Violence would not be limited to the mafia but spray its mischief all over the system. It is exactly to prevent this anarchy that we have, so to speak, invented the state. And again there are counter-arguments: Many crimes take place between equals. Abuses in the compensatory process are not all that probable. Furthermore, in a process of participatory justice, the offender and the victim are not left in limbo. Their discussion must be a public discussion. It would be a discussion where the situation of the victim was scrutinized, where every detail regarding what had happened – legally relevant or not – was brought to the court's attention. Particularly important here would be detailed consideration regarding what could be done for him first and foremost by the offender, secondly by the local neighbourhood, thirdly by the state. Could the harm be compensated, the window repaired, the lock replaced, the wall painted, the loss of time because the car was stolen given back through garden work or washing of the car ten Sundays in a row? Or maybe, once this discussion was started, the damage would not seem so important as it looked in documents written to impress insurance companies? Could physical suffering become slightly less painful through any action on the part of the offender, during days, months or years? And in addition: had the community exhausted all resources that might have offered help? Was it absolutely certain that the local hospital could not do anything? What about a helping hand from the janitor twice a day if the offender took over the cleaning of the basement every Saturday? The situation of the offender would have to be analyzed in the same way. This might expose needs for social, educational, medical or religious action. Not to prevent further crime, but because needs ought to be met.

And to all the objections: why should the impossible cases hinder a decent solution where decency is possible? Why not restrict the area for punishment to the utmost by actively taking away all those cases that might be taken away? Let us construct conciliatory bodies. Let variation blossom when it comes to the selection of personnel, rotation, training, etc. Let us just remember some of the basic lessons from their predecessors: Let us make them vulnerable. Let us not give them power. Let them not become experts. Let them not become distant.

We should have to see it that by and large they were equal to those they had to conciliate and also that they would be living with them. Instead of justice created by a veil of ignorance as suggested by Rawls (1972) this would become justice created through the knowledge that one would have to live with the consequences of the decisions for a long time to come. Such bodies will not be able to handle everything. The state will not wither completely, but will decline a little, one hopes. How far we can go, will be a question of experience. But we cannot move without a goal. The goal must be pain-reduction. Within law as within the other institutions of society. Louk Hulsman once gave a lecture in Oslo with the title: "Penal law as a social problem". From that formulation it follows clearly that the territory of penal law has to be delimited to the utmost extent.

In the long run it will be a question here, as in other main areas in society, of organizing things in such a way that the common people become participants in those matters which are of importance to them instead of just onlookers; or that they become the producers of solutions and not mere consumers. It will be important for us to grope our way forward towards solutions which compel those involved to listen instead of using force, to search for compromise instead of dictates, solutions which encourage compensation instead of reprisals and which, in old-fashioned terms, encourage men to do good instead of, as now, evil.

11.3. Punishment as mourning

There are dangers in the message of civilization of conflicts. This becomes clear if we remember Geoffrey Goorer's analysis of the taboo against mourning. Modern, rational society makes death a modern rational thing. Therefore it also puts a ban on excessive mourning. Anger is no less real than sorrow. It is no less legitimate. Any attempt to civilize conflicts and take pain away might fall under the critique of repressing important elements of life. This book might easily be one more of those taking core activities away from human beings and social systems.

Let me attempt to counteract such an effect by accepting

the expression of immediate anger at the point where mine or other people's rights are hurt. But let us then move one step further. Let us think in analogy with sorrow. If punishments were to be used, they ought to be of a type with important similarities to acts following sorrow. That would establish other important limits to the application of pain:

First, sorrow is to a large extent a *personal matter*. Professionals might take part; the funeral bureau, the priest, maybe some musicians or a chorus. In some cultures, people are hired to express mourning. In Norwegian we called them "*gråtekoner*", that is "weeping ladies". In English they were called "professional mourners". It is an interesting feature of modern life, that these societies, where we use to say that everything has been professionalized, are the very societies where the professional mourners have gone out of business. Modern funerals could very seldom be thought of without those close to the deceased in the centre of the proceedings. When the King dies, State officials would also be in the centre. But in that case, it was the Nation that mourned. When an ordinary person dies, it is still the relatives. In civil court cases, you can hire a representative. Not in funerals, if you are close to the deceased. Either you are there, or you are not.

Secondly, sorrow is an *emotional matter*. Not too much, not too long. But when the coffin disappears in earth or oven, then we are allowed to show emotional strain. Again controlled, but not completely. We are allowed to express grief, and expected to do so. Crocodile tears might be produced at enemies' funerals. But that very performance underlines the legitimacy of the real and natural ones.

Thirdly, mourning is *an act without purpose*. This is right, and of course also completely wrong. Mourning has personal and social functions. Denied access to mourning, people as well as social systems fall into pieces. The expression of grief and sorrow makes continuation possible. We all know. But we do also know that if the expression of sorrow is made with a purpose, then the expression freezes in our throats. This is what makes a state-funeral of a not so loved person into a not so lovely occasion. Sorrow is for the sake of sorrow. This does not prevent us from using sorrow to gain advantages. "You have to stay with me, since I am so sad". Or more common: "If you misbehave, I will be very, very sorry". This is a utilitarian grief, well known through its usefulness, but also despised as a profanation of an emotion known as important to all with something dear to lose.

Loss might lead to sorrow, and mourning. It might also lead to anger, and punishment. There are of course important differences in the process. Mourning does not necessarily have any target, anger converted into punishment has. But there are also similarities. And my point is that the more the anger – expressed through punishment – is given a form with similarities to mourning – the less objectionable I would find the activity. It is a sort of limiting analogy I am attempting to establish. If pain is to be given away, it is only acceptable in a form with structured similarities to mourning.

Concretely: punishments seem more acceptable the more personalized they are, the more emotions they allow for, and the less they are perceived in a utilitarian perspective. If I inflict pain, it must to the largest possible extent be *me,* in emotions, and with pain as the purpose. Not a representative, calm, and with a purpose beyond the expressive one.

What I am describing here, is often classified as an "absolute theory of punishment". Absolute, because no reasons are given. You punish because you punish, just as you are sad because you are sad. An absolute theory of punishment is completely out of fashion among modern penal thinkers. It gives no reason, shows no utility. I like the theory because of that. If there were no purpose behind the pain, it would be more of a clear moral matter. The parties would have to think again and again whether pain was right.

Not whether it was necessary, but right. The chances are great, that the more they thought, the less they would find it right. Reflection would exile anger. The norm-transgressor would be confronted, and might counter-attack. The procedure for punishment would be transformed into a dialogue. We should be back to civil proceedings.

But it is not by chance that absolute theories of punishment are out of fashion, and that the dominant penal theories of our time are of the utilitarian type, with pain as treatment or pain as a deterrent. This is all a true reflection of our societies as often presented to us: Societies of calculating individuals, deeply embedded in the exchange of commodities to maximize individual benefit. We have distant democracy, well suited to a distant penocracy, well suited to serve a large-scale society using taximeters to control the price of all acts. Nothing could be more in harmony with a marked model of exchange than neo-classical thinking around just deserts. A just measure of pain. A proper prize. As we grow more and more international, we will also here establish a world market.

Also in organizational form, our present system of punishment is a pretty good explication of major features of present society. Ours is a society of clients, one where we are represented by others, one where others investigate, debate and decide. Why should we not be clients as victims when we are clients in so many other life spheres? Why should we not let other people receive both money and gratitude to inflict pain on the wrongdoer when we do not really know him, and probably never will. Why should we not buy punishment, when we buy health and happiness?

The reasoning above leads close to the conclusion that punishment as mourning is an impossibility in a society of our type. Which is all right. But also all wrong. We know, all of us, that there is more to our lives than markets and calculation. We have friends for friendship, fall in love for no rational reasons, behave as beasts or heroes even when we know it will not profit us. We talk about markets and calculation, but know pretty well that markets and calculation could not function if there were not a back-stage in operation where words such as communal spirit, totality, solidarity and trust were the important ones. At that back-stage, absolute theories of punishment would probably be a natural feature. Here it would be a question of expressive acts, not goal-oriented ones. It would be punishment as an outcry, not as rational behaviour to take care of something.

In reality, I think that a lot of punishments today have their motivational base at this back-stage. But they are carried out by paid functionaries, which forces theoreticians to give reasons acceptable at the open, utilitaristic front-stage.

When reading or discussing with Andenæs (1950, 1977), Mäkelä (1975) and their followers, I do increasingly get the feeling that we might find common ground if we all dared to embark on a debate on solidarity, social demands, cohesion and other elements which made a society into more than the sum of individuals and rational acts. Advocates for general prevention have – and more so than advocates for treatment – important sociological elements behind their reasoning: We might sometimes be able to create doubts concerning the general preventive effects of a certain type of punishment. But we will seldom be able to convince the believer, because behind the general preventive idea is another idea, one that says that something has to happen when wrongs have occurred, something in analogy with mourning. In other words, many arguments in favour of pain delivery as a necessity for general prevention or deterrence, might be elements of an absolute theory of punishment in disguise.

These views must not be pushed too far. Theories of general prevention or deterrence have to be evaluated on the basis of their own stated merits, and in the extreme versions such as removing all police or imposing death sentences for traffic offences, they have obvious merits. All I suggest, is that there is more behind some parts of the claims for punishment than stated in the simplistic, utilitarian version. And it is important to get that "more" out into the open, make it explicit, and start a debate on it. Pain delivered as a measure of general prevention can be controlled in a neo-classical system of justice. But as argued earlier, this is a primitive system of control with unwanted side effects. If at least parts of the activities are related to an absolute theory of punishment, this might open the way for new discussions of the needs for pain, and of forms of control of the pain. Our situation is one where incentives for "an absolute type of punishment" are transformed into a system suited for handling utilitarian punishments. This leads to a perpetual dissatisfaction with law and order in society. The *gesellschaft*-structure or market-structure of society is cared for, but the *gemeinschaft*-structure is undernourished. Within penal law, this leads to an ever-lasting demand for more punishments carried out by representatives who – rightly in the impossible situation in which they are placed – perceive themselves as a buffer between a savage population filled with a lust for vengance, and some misfits in need of protection against receiving too much pain. This situation adds to a basic instability in societies of our type.

What then, are the consequences of this analysis?

Let me suggest two.

First, pain delivery in western society is *not* carried out in a form with structural similarities to mourning. It is motivated by anger, *but expressed through representation.* This explains probably why the volume of pain delivery can vary so much from time to time, and between societies. The amount – as well as the activity in general – is not so closely linked to the informal web of interaction within western societies that variation in volume matters. The paid representatives – judges, prison officers, prison administrators, parole directors – build up various systems for pain delivery. In this process they are of course influenced by numerous reasons other than those related to any calculation of which volume of pain delivery would be the "right one". But this means at the same time that we would be more free to work for a reduction in the volume of pain delivery within the framework of certain forms of absolute theories of punishment.

Secondly, if punishment were to be accepted, it would have to be of the expressive type related to mourning. Then a whole row of new questions would have to be raised: Was the punishment one where ordinary people – including the victim – took part in all aspects of the decision? Did they take part in the actual execution of the punishment? Did they all – one after the other – carry out the work inside the penal establishments? How much did *everybody* in society know about all the details? What could be done to increase knowledge? Might local TV be brought into local courts and punishment institutions all over the country? If one hesitated to bring in local TV, ought they not instead to hesitate to bring in punishment? If pain is too bad to be executed by everybody, and seen by everybody, is it not because it is too bad? If the purpose of pain was pain, was it then arranged so that this became crystal clear to everybody.

If we brought it close, we would become participants, sometimes accomplices. That would be when it did not feel right, when we, for example, knew the offender, or the victim, or the situation or similar situations and saw that this was not a case where pain was right. It would create an opening for that fundamental discussion of moral matters where norm-clarification would become the central task.

But with these new questions, and bearing in mind those conditions discussed in Chapter 10, we are probably able to see that absolute theories of punishments in a society based on participation and not representation, might easily lead to a society of pain-reduction. It is absolute theories of punishment disguised as utilitarian which in a society of representatives creates the strong incentives towards using pain. An absolute theory, seen as absolute, and executed by those close to the scene of misbehaviour, would not by any necessity have the same effect. An absolute theory of punishment, applied between equals standing close to each other, would in this concrete application most probably be converted into a civil conflict.

11.4. The informal economy

This book is not based on any belief that ideas change the world. Not ideas alone. But ideas might help to change it, when other conditions are right.

Are they?

There are some obvious needs for experts on behaviour control in a society like ours. Several complexities of our time are of a magnitude that cannot be handled by ordinary people in ordinary, fragmented social systems. There are also enormously powerful centralizing forces in operation, particularly fostered through the military establishments and by the effects of international organizations for trade and industry. Participatory justice becomes unreal if societies, to make ready for catastrophe, become organized in a monolithic pattern, where action is based on orders, not choice, and where any experiment is seen as dangerous living in an equilibrium based on brinkmanship.

But there are also other forces in operation. I described some of them in Chapter 9.3. as subterranean patterns, and in 9.4. as counter cultures. Let us now move one step further.

Exactly half of the Norwegian population belongs to the work force, in the meaning of having paid work. The other half is outside, provided for in some form or another. And it is that latter half which is on the increase, in Norway as in all highly industrialized countries.

Stepwise, we have in countries of this sort been through four important stages. First, *the primary sector* – farming and fishing – has become mechanized. The number of hands needed has gone down dramatically. That was good for *the secondary sector* represented by industry. That sector got more competing empty hands, until their level of mechanization reached an unbelievably high level, and their need for workers also diminished. Again good for *the third sector* – service, administration, hospitals, universities, which happily absorbed some of the surplus – until the vengeance from the up to now unindustrialized countries reached us. This is what has just happened. Those societies still in the second and third stage have entered the by now close to completely open market, taken over essential parts of production and left us with a huge service sector to be paid for by the diminishing returns from our national industrial system. At this stage, most highly industrial countries have chosen the same instinctive reaction; they stop the growth of the service sector. Those countries worst off start to diminish that sector also. The post-industrial society is there.

This is not the place for a thorough analysis of this whole development. But what happens has consequences for social control. The whole industrial system is in a process of dramatic change. This is bound to have consequences for the ways people will relate.

For our purposes, it seems useful to describe separately the effects on two major categories; those with paid work, and the other half, that is those without. For the first category, the major effect of relevance to us is the simple fact that he/she will gradually receive less of everything through official salary. The bargaining power is broken. Her or his firm will have to compete with a firm in Korea, in

Thailand, in Tanzania. At the same time direct or indirect taxes will increase, and/or the costs of all sorts of public service will increase. It cannot be otherwise, when fewer people within production have to pay for more people outside. The total effects will be diminished returns from officially paid work.

Paid workers get less. At the same time it becomes less common to have an ordinary paid job at all. Unemployment is on a dramatic increase within nearly all countries in the old industrialized world.

So far is common knowledge. And what follows, ought to have been, since it is obvious: Unemployment does not mean that people stop working. To the surprise of some, it becomes clear that there exist other forms of labour than the officially registered one. People lose their employment, but continue to work. Behind the official labour-market is a grey one for the unemployed and for those with insufficient income. Since taxes are so high, the mechanic will fix his friend's car in the evening, sometimes for money, often for nothing that same evening, but then for some return service another day. They are not alone in doing this. As Gershuny (1979) and Pahl (1980), and also the two in combination (1980), have pointed out in stimulating articles, there exists an economy behind the official one, parts of it legal, parts of it half-legal, and parts solidly illegal. This informal economy is growing as a result of the shrinkage of the official economy. There exist behaviour-patterns and exchange relationships with a remarkable resemblance to forms in existence before the industrial revolution. The famous poachers of England are still vividly alive, and vegetables are happily being produced in the back-yards – for exchange with other non-taxable utilities. As the official rate of unemployment increases in western societies, these informal economic activities are bound to increase in importance. We get two economies. One official, within highly automatized plants and with a taxable profit, which provides a base for a minimum of social security of the type we know today. But in addition, we get the informal one.

By informal economy, I mean something different from what Ivan Illich (1981) calls shadow work. Shadow work is to Illich what has to be done to keep the industrially employed going. It is the wife needed to keep the husband able to go to the factory. But Illich contrasts shadow work with vernacular values or "folk"-values. And that is closer to my theme. The formal economy as we know it through labour-contracts, salaries, tax-deductions, job safety and all those regulations accomplished through centuries of labour actions is for an increasing number of western workers just becoming a non-reality. The plant is moved to Korea or Thailand and the Western worker is back to a situation with provocative similarities to his distant past.

This new, and very old, situation is bound to have consequences for social organization, and thereby for social control. As Pahl (1980) in particular has pointed out, the situation is one where some of the more handicapped groups within the old industrialized societies suddenly might have a particular advantage:

Those categories or strata which have resisted most effectively incorporation into the dominant values of industrial capitalism may be able to survive the problems imposed by the decline of formal employment in the years ahead more easily.

Pahl specifies three groups of unemployed, with those most advantaged at the top:

1. Those with skills and services available for sale or for exchange and who have the local knowledge and contacts to provide access to informal markets.
2. Those with few or no tradeable skills or products but who have access to local networks and have the resources to buy such skills and facilities that they need.

3. Those who have neither skills, knowledge or resources to contribute to the informal economy. In terms of a more traditional system of stratification such a disadvantaged category might fall in the middle of the social hierarchy, being the petty bourgeoisie with some clerical or minor bureaucratic or managerial administrative skill and which has been geographically and possibly also socially mobile. They are isolated from communal resources and do not have enough surplus income to buy their way in.

In other words: it pays to be a member. If the formal economy deteriorates even further, membership will be a necessity for survival. We are anew in the situation most humans always have been in, where participation, trust, communal living and mutual dependence become the central elements in life. These are exactly the conditions where participatory justice might function at its best.

11.5. Justice to the weak?

And what then about weak parties not getting their rights? Oppressed wives whom a board of neighbours did not dare to stand up for, minorities met with prejudice at the local clinic, a clinic the board members might depend on in the future, appartments where children are heard crying constantly, but where no one dare break into the castle of privacy. Would not participatory justice make weak parties even more weak than they are today?

It depends.

Ordinary professionally staffed criminal courts might function as a protective device and bring justice to the weak if:
– the society was one of inequality with regard to power, but with ideals that weak parties ought to be protected.
– and if the rulers as well as their courts took great care to activate the protective devices.
– and if the society was a transparent one where abuses were easily registered.
– and if the weak parties trusted the courts.

– and if the courts were open to all sorts of complaints, and acted according to the ideals.

This would of course still be a justice accepting the basic inequalities making the weak parties just weak. It would be that the husband should not beat his wife more than she deserved, that blacks should not be arrested for walking through a white community when they had a task to perform there. It is better than nothing, but not quite as much as often stated. But let me repeat it, just to protect the obvious from oblivion; independent courts do represent an important source for the protection of weak parties against abuses of the minimum rights ascribed them.

This then raises important questions on how to accomplish a greater extent of participatory justice, without losing important protective devices within our recent system. Is it possible to construct some sort of neighbourhood justice with the advantages of participation, but without losing the protection of legality? Can the State come in and help the weak parties in a conflict, but help them without taking over the conflict? And what happens when the State itself is one of the parties? Again, any answer to this must of course take into consideration the weak position weak parties have within our existing system.

A related question is how to prevent ideas of civilization and participation from becoming perverted. Recent experiences with "alternatives to prison" indicate that they easily turn into "additions to prison", and that conditional sentences in reality turn into more time spent in prison. The lesson from periods of "treatment for crime" ought also to be kept vividly in mind. If pain delivery is limited, will we then get a rehearsal of the old story? Will new, subtle punishment appear, administered within these seemingly so civil bodies. Sceptics will be greatly needed. So also will independent research, institutionally as well as intellectually protected against embracement by authorities.

This book is not a book on revolution, it is one on reform. Essential questions are whether courts can be more participatory, or whether bodies for conflict handling can be added to the recent structure. A central concern here is to attempt to activate neighbourhoods, which again will make it more known, to the participants, what actually goes on within them. As Ray Shonholtz has expressed it (private communication) on the basis of his experience with community boards in San Francisco, weak parties will generally have a better chance if neigbourhoods become more neighbourly. Maltreatment of wife or children is more easy to hide if the whole family is hidden, than if wife and children have many contacts in the community. Kinberg, Inghe and Riemer (1943) illustrated vividly how this factor operated in cases of father-daughter incest. In isolated families, the father's physical dominance got out of control. Community integration gives weak parties within sub-systems a chance of making their misery known, and also of establishing protective coalitions. If weak parties were to gain, one should probably see to it that the relevant system was not too small, not so small that coalitions were impossible – and not too large – not so large that transparency was impossible. I share the feeling of relief and freedom by being among strangers. I am aware of the blessings of a community without community character. But I am afraid there are others who pay the bill.

But of course, integration does not always help. Neighbourhoods might organize *against* minorities. Participatory justice might thus mean increased strength to the oppressor. This raises enormously complex problems that I will not go into, except for two remarks. First, few among us would claim that to work for a "non-community" would be a good solution. The problem then seems more to be how closely knit a neighbourhood one should work for, and not an all or nothing. Living in post-industrial society of the Norwegian type, my simplistic view would be: More than at present. In danger of falling into the ditch on one side of the road, one can easily argue for steering more towards the other side, even without knowing exactly how far out that other dangerous ditch is.

Strengthening participatory justice would, however, clearly strengthen tendencies to pay tribute to local values. Justice would not be quite as equal from neighbourhood to neighbourhood as it is supposed to be today. Participatory justice will in other words. strengthen the survival ability of local values. In a world-perspective, that might be a considerable gain. Our highly industrialized world is increasingly creating one homogeneous culture of consumers. Subcultures, native populations, completely other ways of thinking and acting, all this has probably become exterminated to a greater extent during the last 30 years than ever before in the history of our globe. Diversity in social arrangements has become heavily reduced. But we know that diversity often functions as a protection of a species. Some among us looking at the highly military, industrial establishments in East and West as a threat against alternative values and actions, would perceive the fostering of diversity as being of extreme importance. States nearly always defend themselves through armour similar to that of their greatest perceived enemies. Neighbourhoods might succeed by being so small that they are not worth conquering, so different that they are difficult to digest, so cohesive that they through joint action can force giants to find other areas for the contaminating plant, alternative areas which also turn out to be cohesive and resistant. In this broader perspective, participatory justice might turn out to be one of the essential elements in the protection of diversity, and thereby also of values in danger of extermination.

If these views have any validity, then the major tasks ahead of us are not a discussion of crime control. Nor are ney a discussion of theories of treatment, deterrence, or types of punishment. The major task will instead be one of discussion on how to establish a social system that provides the utmost possibilities for exposure and discussion of the total set of values in society. How can we create systems that ensure that all important values, and all important parties, are included in the considerations? How can we arrange it so that the conflict-setting mechanisms themselves, through their organization, reflect the type of society we should like to see reflected and help this type of society come into being?

11.6. Limits to limits?

Could it ever happen? Could we imagine social systems where the parties by and large relied on civil solutions? Would there not always occur cases where someone demanded that punishment had to be carried out?

Two potential cases of such demands are particularly important.

The first is the case of the vengeful victim. The offender has hurt my body. Nothing, except revenge on the offender's body, can restore the situation. Let us imagine that this was the victim's reasoning. Let us also imagine that compensation had been attempted, and that the situation was one of equality of power, vulnerability, and mutual dependence between the parties. If in this situation the victim still insisted on revenge, should not she or he then rightfully be allowed to inflict pain on the offender if she or he so dared?

To this question the first answer must be a moral one. In a system accepting revenge, the victim or his or her representatives would have the right to retaliate. In a system emphasizing the value of forgiveness, the victim would be encouraged to turn the other cheek to the malefactor.

But if the victim does forgive, a new question emerges.

Should the victim in all cases be allowed to show kindness, to forgive? What about serious crimes, so upsetting to the surrounding community that they – the surrounders – insisted that pain had to be used. The mother of the murdered child forgave the offender, but the surroundings did not. Who should be listened to?

This would, in the concrete cases, depend on what sort of system the parties were members of. If the system consisted of victim and offender, and only these two, the problem would be non-existent, at least for these two. But the more members the system had, and the less closely related the victim and/or the offender was to the other members, the greater the problem of community reaction would become.

Rudolf Steiner (1972) has introduced a useful analogy between language and a sense of justice. We are all born with a potentiality for talking. But we do not acquire a language unless we associate with other humans. Likewise we are born with a potential sense of justice. But we do not build it up before we associate with other humans. It is through interaction that we build up a sense of what is right language as well as a sense of what is the right answer to deviance. Sense of language as well as sense of justice are thus social products.

In both cases, the sense of right – in language or morality – can be influenced from sources far away. The Queen of Spain established a grammar for correct language. Illegitimate language was kept under contol. Thereby also illegitimate thoughts (Illich 1981). The same is the case within law. State law is the grammar. The ideal type of participatory justice would be one based on the participants' own sense of justice – their legal local dialect. The more the rules are laid down by the State, the greater are the chances that agreements between parties will not suffice – as seen from the State's point of view.

In Chapter 10, I have described some conditions for a low level of pain infliction. It will be recalled that my general hypothesis was that social systems organized according to these principles would also exhibit great hesitancy in their application of pain. But at the same time, State government will most often represent a negation of these principles. In other words; the more State, the more the conditions are laid down for punishment, and the less State, the less the conditions encourage punishment.

But here the reasoning brings us into a dilemma. In a small, stable system the chances are great that the sense of justice will be shared by all the participants. They talk the same legal language. This means that the victim's forgiveness will be the other system-members' forgiveness as well. But what if that did not happen? Individual cases might deviate from the pattern. A deviant victim might be in favour of torture, or a subsystem might believe in it. To control such cases, we need large systems with independent non-vulnerable State power – in other words exactly the social conditions that I have suggested create possiblities of using pain in social relations. To control cruelty, we might need more State power. But creating State power might lead to more use of pain. I see no way out of the dilemma in principle. The nearest I can come to an answer is to say: so little State as we dare. So small systems as we dare. So independent systems as we dare. So egalitarian systems as we dare. So vulnerable participants as we dare. In such cases, they would be inhibited in using pain. But I have then no answer to the question of what to do with a phenomenon such as, for example, pain application which seems "natural" to system-members. Maybe there exists an optimum somewhere, some "five grains of State-power"?

But in practical politics, I have an answer. Our time is the heyday of the large national States. They are seen as natural solutions rather than problem-creating ones. Since that is such an overwhelming tendency, any move in the opposite direction must be a right one. The situation where the punitive consequences of too little State will emerge are so far away that any concrete advice in our recent situation would be to work towards the opposite principle for social organization.

Chapter 12. In contrast to pain

This is a book on pain. But nowhere has it here been stated what pain is. It is also a book on social systems. Therefore, barely do we meet human beings except as system-members. Browsing through the pages, I miss a point of orientation above Hell, a point expressed in the longings of human beings. C. S. Lewis (1940) has described such a point. It is high time that criminology pay more attention to heaven, so let me end this little book by quoting Lewis on the negation of pain (pp 133–135):

You may have noticed that the books you really love are bound together by a secret thread. You know very well what is the common quality that makes you love them, though you cannot put it into words: but most of your friends do not see it at all, and often wonder why, liking this, you should also like that. Again, you have stood before some landscape, which seems to embody what you have been looking for all your life; and then turned to the friend at your side who appears to be seeing what you saw – but at the first words a gulf yawns between you, and you realise that this landscape means something totally different to him, that he is pursuing an alien vision and cares nothing for the ineffable suggestion by which you are transported. Even in your hobbies, has there not always been some secret attraction which the others are curiously ignorant of – something, not to be identified with, but always on the verge of breaking through, the smell of cut wood in the workshop or the clap-clap of water against the boat's side? Are not all lifelong friendships born at the moment when at last you meet another human being who has some inkling (but faint and uncertain even in the best) of that something which you were born desiring, and which, beneath the flux of other desires and in all the momentary silences between the louder passions, night and day, year by year, from childhood to old age, you are looking for, watching for, listening for? You have never *had* it. All the things that have ever deeply possessed your soul have been but hints of it – tantalising glimpses, promises never quite fulfilled, echoes that died away just as they caught your ear. But if it should really become manifest – if there ever came an echo that did not die away but swelled into the sound itself – you would know it. Beyond all possibility of doubt you would say "Here at last is the thing I was made for". We cannot tell each other about it. It is the secret signature of each soul, the incommunicable and unappeasable want, the thing we desired before we met our wives or made our friends or chose our work, and which we shall still desire on our deathbeds, when the mind no longer knows wife or friend or work. While we are, this is. If we lose this, we lose all.

Bibliography

Alternativer til frihedsstraf – Et debatoplæg. (Alternatives to imprisonment – a debate proposal.) Betænkning nr. 806, København 1977.

American friend's service committee: *Struggle for justice*. N. Y. 1971.

Andenæs, Johs: Almenprevensjonen – illusjon eller realitet? (General prevention – illusion or reality.) *Nordisk tidsskrift for kriminalvidenskab* 1950, 33, 103–133.

Andenæs, Johs: *Punishment and deterrence*. With a foreword by Norval Morris. Ann Arbor 1974.

Anttila, Inkeri: Konservativ och radikal kriminalpolitik i Norden. (Conservative and radical criminal policy within the Nordic countries). *Nordisk tidsskrift for kriminalvidenskab* 1967, *55*, 237–251.

Anttila, Inkeri: Et förslag til strafflagsreform i Finland. (A proposal for penal reform in Finland.) *Nordisk tidsskrift for kriminalvidenskab* 1977, 65, 102–106.

Aubert, Vilhelm: *Om straffens sosiale funksjoner*. (On the social functions of punishment.) Oslo 1954.

Aubert, Vilhelm: Legal justice and mental health. *Psychiatry*, 1958, *21*, 101–113.

Aubert, Vilhelm and Thomas Mathiesen: Forbrytelse og sykdom. (Crime and Illness.) *Tidsskrift for samfunnsforskning* 1962, *3*, pp 169–93.

Balvig, Flemming: Om ældre kvinders angst for kriminalitet. (On elderly women's fear of criminality.) *Rapport fra kontaktseminariet, Sundvolden, Norge 1979. Scandinavian Research Council for Criminology*. pp. 132–139.

Beccaria, Cesare: *Dei deilitti e delle pene. Om brott och straff*. Livorno 1766, Stockholm–Roma 1977, 203 p.

Becker, Howard: Whose side are we on? *Social problems*, 1967, *14*, 239–247.

Bianchi, Herman: Het assensusmodel – Een studie over het binnenlands asylrecht. *Tijdschrift voor criminologie*, 1979, *21*, pp. 167–179. In Norwegian: Assensusmodellen. En studie over innenlandsk asylrett. Stensilserien, *Institutt for kriminologi og strafferett*, Oslo 1981.

Bjørkan, Wendy: Lensmannsetaten: En overlevning fra fortiden eller en modell for fremtiden? (The sheriff – a relic from the past or a model for the future?) *Institutt for kriminologi og strafferett, 1977, nr. 25* Mimeo.

Bondeson, Ulla: *Fången i fångsamhället*. (The prisoner within the society of captives.) Malmö 1974.

Bottoms, A. E.: An introduction to "The coming crisis". In: Bottoms, A. E. and R. H. Preston: *The coming penal crisis. A criminological and theological exploration*. Edinburgh 1980.

Brottsförebyggande rådet: Nytt straffsystem. Ideer och förslag. Stockholm. Rapport 1977:7 (Also published in English Summary: The National Swedish

119

Council for crime prevention: A new penal system. Ideas and proposals, Stockholm 1978, Report No 5.)

Börjeson, Bengt: *Om påföljders verkningar.* (On the effects of sanctions.) Uppsala, 1966.

Callewaert, Staf and Bengt An. Nilsson: *Samhället, skolan och skolans indre arbete.* (Society, the school and the work inside the school.) Sweden 1979.

Christiansen, Karl O., Mogens Moe and Leif Senholt, in collaboration with Ken Schubell, and Karin Zedeler: *Effektiviteten af forvaring og særfængsel m.v.* (The effectiveness of non-penal incarceration and special prison etc.) Denmark 1972. Statens trykningskontor, Betænkning nr. 644.

Christie, Nils: *Tvangsarbeid og alkoholbruk.* (Forced labour and the use of alcohol.) Oslo 1960 a.

Christie, Nils: Reaksjonenes virkninger. (The effects of the sanctions.) *Nordisk tidsskrift for kriminalvidenskab* 1960 b, *49*, pp 129–144.

Christie, Nils: Forskning om individual-prevensjon kontra almenprevensjon. (Research on individual prevention versus general prevention.) *Lov og Rett* 1971, nr. X, 49–60.

Christie, Nils: *Fangevoktere i konsentrasjonsleire.* (Guards in concentration camps.) Oslo 1972.

Christie, Nils: Conflicts as Property. *Br.j. Crim*, 1977, *17*, 1–19.

Clarke, Bill: *Enough room for joy. Jean Vanier's L'Arche.* A message for our time. London 1974.

Cohen, Stan: Guilt, justice and tolerance: Some old concepts for a new criminology. 1977, Mim. *Dept. of sociology, Univ. of Essex, England.*

Cohen, Stan: The Punitive City: Notes on the Dispersal of Social Control, *Contemporary Crises,* 1979, *3*, pp. 339–64.

Cohen, Stan and Laurie Taylor: *Psychological survival. The experience of long-term imprisonment.* G.B. 1972.

Cooper, L.et.al.: *The iron fist and the velvet glove: An analysis of the U.S. police.* Berkeley 1974.

Dahl, Tove Stang: Statsmakt og sosial kontroll. (State power and social control.) In Rune Slagstad, ed: *Om Staten.* Oslo 1977.

Dahl, Tove Stang: *Barnevern og samfunnsvern.* (Child welfare and social defence) Oslo 1978.

Dalgard, Odd Steffen: *Abnorme lovovertredere. Diagnose og prognose.* (Abnormal offenders, Diagnosis and prognosis.) Oslo 1966.

Ehrlich, Isaac: The Deterrent Effect of Capital Punishment. A Question of Life and Death. *Am Ec. Rev.* 1975, *65*, pp. 397–417.

Englund, G. och Hasselakollektivet: *Tvånget til frihet.* (Compulsive freedom.) Stockholm 1978.

Eriksson, Lars: *Varning för vård.* (Warning against treatment.) 1967.

Foucault, Michel: *Surveiller et punir.* France 1975. (Discipline and punish. London 1978.)

Gershuny, J. I.: The informal economy. Its role in post-industrial society. *Futures,* 1979, *12*, pp. 3–15.

Gershuny, J. I. and R. E. Pahl: Work outside employment: some preliminary speculations. *New universities quarterly,* 1980, *34*, pp. 120–135.

Gluckman, Max: *The judicial process among the Barotse of Northern Rhodesia.* Manchester 1967.

Goldschmidt, Verner: Den grøndlanske kriminallov og dens sociologiske baggrund. (The criminal law of Greenland and its sociological background.) *Nordisk tidsskrift for kriminal videnskab*, 1954, *42*, pp. 133–148 and 242–268.

Gorer, Geoffrey: *Death, grief and mourning in contemporary Britain.* N.Y. 1965.

Gottfredson, Don, Leslie T. Wilkins and Peter B. Hoffman: *Guidelines for parole and sentencing. A policy control method,* USA 1978.

Gouldner, Al: The sociologist as partisan. Sociology and the welfare state. *The American Sociologist,* 1968, 3, 103–116.

Greenberg, David F. and Drew Humphries: The cooptation of fixed sentencing reform. *Crime and delinquency* 1980, *26*, pp. 206 –225.

Hernes, Gudmund and Knud Knudsen: *Utdanning og ulikhet.* (Education and inequality.) NOU 1976:46.

Hirsch, Andrew von: Prediction of criminal conduct and preventive confinement of convicted persons. *Buffalo law review,* 1972, *21*, pp. 717–758.

Hirsch, Andrew von: *Doing justice.* Report of the committee for the study of incarceration. N. Y. 1976.

Homans, George Caspar: *The human group.* London 1951.

Ignatieff, Michael: *A just measure of pain. The penitentiary in the industrial revolution 1750–1850.* G. B. 1978.

Illich, Ivan: *The right to useful unemployment and its professional enemies.* London 1978.

Illich, Ivan: *Shadow work.* Boston – London 1981.

Jakobsen, Knut Dahl: Politisk fattigdom. (Political poverty.) *Kontrast* 1964, *3*, pp. 5–11.

Kinberg, Olof, Gunnar Inghe and Svend Riemer: *Incest problemet i Sverige* (The incest problem in Sweden.) Stockholm 1943.

Kutschinsky, Berl: *Law, pornography and crime: The Danish experience.* London, in press (1981).

Lewis, C. S.: *The problem of pain,* Great Britain 1940. Fontana books 1980.

Lindblom, Ulf. Smärtbehandling under omprövning (Treatment of pain reconsidered.) *Nordisk medisin* 1980, *95,* p. 75.

Lusseyrand, Jacques: *And there was light.* Boston 1963. (Norwegian edition: *Og det ble lys.* Dreyer 1978.)

Madsen, Børge: I skorpionens halespids. Et speciale om mig og Christiania (In the tail of the scorpion.) *Christiania* 1979.

Mathiesen, Thomas: *The politics of abolition. Essays in political action theory.* Scandinavian studies in criminology. Oslo and London 1974.

Mathiesen, Thomas: *Den skjulte disiplinering* (The hidden discipline.) Oslo 1978.

Milgram, Stanley: Some conditions of obedience and disobedience to authority. *Human relations,* 1965, *18,* pp. 57–75.

Myrdal, Jan: Folket och ordningen (The people and the order). *Folket i Bild/ Kulturfront.* Stockholm 1977. 6 nb. 4, 9 and 15.

Mäkelä, Klaus: Om straffens verkningar. (On the effects of punishments.) *Eripainos oikeustiede* 1975, *6,* 237–280.

Neznansky, Friedrich: New information on Soviet criminal statistics. (An insider's report.) Paper presented at the annual meeting of *the American Society of Criminology,* 1979.

Olaussen, Leif Petter: *Fordeling og utvikling av forbrytelser i Norge 1957–75.* (Distribution and developments of crime in Norway 1957–1975.)

121

Hovedoppgave i kriminologi. Institutt for kriminologi og strafferett. 1979.

Pahl, R. E., Employment, work and the domestic division of labour. *Int. of Urban and Regional research*, 1980, *4*, pp. 1–20.

Parmann, Øistein ed: *Vidaråsen landsby. Ideer, dagligliv, bakgrunn.* (Vidaråsen village. Ideas, daily life, background.) Oslo 1980.

Platt, Anthon *The Child Savers. The invention of delinquency,* Chicago 1969.

Radzinowicz _eon: *Ideology and Crime.* N. Y. 1966.

Ramsøy, Natalie Rogoff: *Sosial mobilitet i Norge.* (Social mobility in Norway.) Oslo 1977.

Rawls, John: *A theory of justice.* Oxford 1972.

Roszak, Teodore: *The making of a counter culture. Reflections on the technocratic society and its youthful opposition.* N. Y. 1969.

Sellin, Thorsten: *Capital punishment.* N. Y. 1967.

Snare, Annika: Konfliktlösare i närmiljön. (Conflikt solution in the local milieu.) *Rapport fra 21 nordiske forskerseminar på Lillehammer, Norge 1979, Scandinavian Research Council for Criminology.* pp. 32–79.

Stang, Hans Jakob: *Mangelfullt utviklede og/eller varig svekkede sjelsevner. Diagnoser og prognoser.* (Limited or lastingly diminished mental abilities. Diagnosis and prognosis.) Oslo 1966.

Stortingsmelding nr. 104 (1977–78) *Om kriminalpolitikken.* Oslo 1978. (Parliamentary report no 104. Concerning criminal policy.)

Straffrättskommittens betänkande 1976:72. Band 1 og 2, 1978. (Consideration of the Penal Law Committee 1976:72) Helsinki 1978.

Strindberg, August: *Tjänstekvinnans son.* (The maid-servant's son) Stockholm 1878.

Støkken, Anne Marie og medarbeidere: *Politiet i det norske samfunnet.* (The police in the Norwegian society.) Oslo 1974.

Sykes, Gresham M.: *The society of captives. A study of a maximum security prison.* USA 1958.

Takala, Hannu: Den klassiska straffrättens renässans. *Utskrift av innlegg på seminar avholdt av Nordisk Samarbeidsråd for Kriminologi, Kiljava, Finland 1978.* 11 s.

The twentieth century fund task force on criminal sentencing: *Fair and certain punishment.* USA 1976.

Thelander, Anna: *Hassela kollektivet. En rapport om vårdinnehåll och vårdideologi på et hem för unge narkomaner.* (The Hassela collectivity.) Stockholm 1979.

Valen-Senstad: *For lov og rett i 200 år. Oslo Politis historie.* (For law and order in 200 years. The history of the Oslo-police.) Oslo 1953.

Wheeler, Stanton. *Controlling delinquents.* N. Y. 1968.

EINSTEIN
the
PENGUIN

Books by Iona Rangeley

EINSTEIN THE PENGUIN

EINSTEIN THE PENGUIN: THE CASE OF THE FISHY DETECTIVE

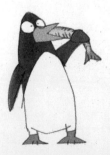

Iona Rangeley

EINSTEIN the PENGUIN

Illustrated by David Tazzyman

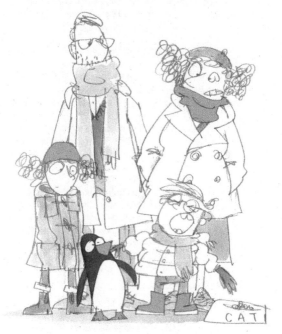

HarperCollins *Children's Books*

First published in the United Kingdom by
HarperCollins *Children's Books* in 2021
Published in this edition in 2022
HarperCollins *Children's Books* is a division of HarperCollins*Publishers* Ltd
1 London Bridge Street
London SE1 9GF

www.harpercollins.co.uk

HarperCollins*Publishers*
Macken House, 39/40 Mayor Street Upper
Dublin 1, D01 C9W8, Ireland

5

Text copyright © Iona Rangeley 2021
Illustrations copyright © David Tazzyman 2021
Cover illustrations copyright © David Tazzyman 2021
Cover design copyright © HarperCollins*Publishers* Ltd 2022
All rights reserved

ISBN 978–0–00–847599–4

Iona Rangeley and David Tazzyman assert the moral right to be identified as the author
and illustrator of the work respectively.
A CIP catalogue record for this title is available from the British Library.

Typeset in Arno Pro Regular 13pt/24pt
Printed and bound in the UK using 100% renewable electricity
at CPI Group (UK) Ltd

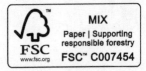

*To my parents, even though they never let me
have my own penguin*

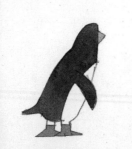

CHAPTER ONE

London Zoo

It was a very long time ago now, as long ago as last Christmas, that the Stewarts first met Einstein.

It was a cold sort of Christmas. The sort where days end early and forget to start on time, and the fairy lights out in the street don't quite make up for the darkness.

'What can we do with the children?' said Mrs Stewart to her husband one Saturday towards the beginning of December. The early afternoon was bitterly chilly, and no one had found the heart to venture out into it yet. 'We don't want them to get too bored. Imogen might paint the cat again.'

Mr Stewart sighed into his tea and turned a page of his newspaper. 'She's grown out of that sort of thing, hasn't she?'

'I don't know,' said Mrs Stewart. 'Maybe.'

The children, at that precise moment in time, were keeping themselves busy in the sitting room. Arthur, who was six, was drawing pictures in a notebook while Imogen, his big sister, was sitting cross-legged in the corner, fiddling with the dials on a radio. Occasionally it would make a crackling sound and then stop again, and she would triumphantly declare to her brother that she had 'fixed it'.

'Maybe we should take them to the zoo!' said Mrs Stewart suddenly.

'The zoo?' Mr Stewart repeated.

'Yes!' said Mrs Stewart, who had spotted an advertisement on the back of her husband's newspaper.

'Arthur might like to draw the animals!'

Mr Stewart frowned into the article he was reading. He rather liked the idea of going to the zoo. It was exciting: maybe he'd see a lion! 'Well, all right,' he said eventually, in a careful sort of voice. 'If you think the children will enjoy it.'

'Imogen! Arthur!' Mrs Stewart called, and Imogen came skidding into the kitchen on the slippery tiles. Her brother followed calmly a few moments later. 'Get your shoes and coats on. We're going to the zoo.'

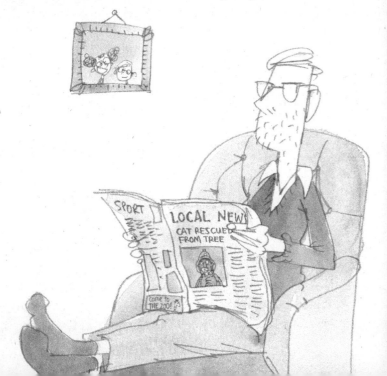

'The zoo?' said Arthur.

'Yes. As a treat. It's very cold outside, so wrap up warm. Imogen, where's your jumper? You haven't lost it again, have you?'

Several minutes of rushing about the house passed. Imogen's jumper was retrieved from the cat, and three separate arguments were had about scarves. By the time they stepped outside and made their way

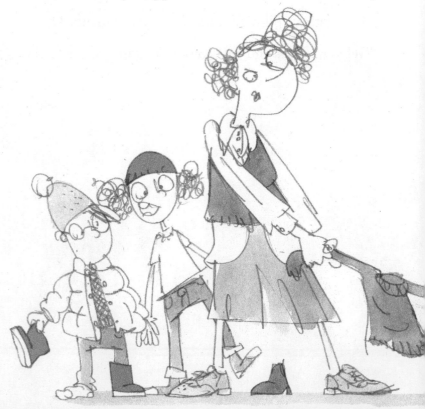

towards the bus stop, the sky had gone through a whole new shade of grey, and the sun – no doubt a little bored of waiting – had hidden itself behind the tall trees on the edge of Hampstead Heath.

'It's cold,' said Imogen, reluctantly taking her father's hand as they crossed the road.

'I *did* tell you to put a scarf on, darling,' said Mrs Stewart, who was just a bit ahead of them.

'My scarf is *pink*!' said Imogen. 'I don't *like* pink any more!'

'She's nine, you know, Rachel,' said Mr Stewart through a smile. 'Very grown-up.'

The bus was a Saturday afternoon sort of busy, bustling with shopping bags and umbrellas. There weren't enough seats for everyone, so Arthur sat on

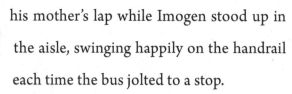

his mother's lap while Imogen stood up in the aisle, swinging happily on the handrail each time the bus jolted to a stop.

When they got off, the sky was greyer still, and there were leaves blowing in the cold wind as they walked alongside the canal.

There is something about chilly afternoons that makes people all the more determined to enjoy themselves, and the Stewarts weren't the only family in London who had thought the zoo might be a sensible place to spend their teatime: it was very busy.

The children were immediately anxious to examine all the sweets in the gift-shop window, while Mr Stewart – having had a brief panic about whether he'd lost his wallet – found it and went to buy tickets.

'Right, where to first?' he said, returning a moment later with a map.

Imogen declared that she wanted to see a polar bear, and make friends with it.

'I don't think they have polar bears,' said Mrs Stewart, taking the map from her husband. 'Why don't we wander past the monkeys and finish up at the penguins?'

Imogen pursed her lips and frowned, but the idea of monkeys was a good one, and she quickly cheered up. After a few moments, *both* of her parents were having to shout at her to slow down.

'Where does *that* monkey come from?' said Arthur, clutching his father's arm at the sight of a particularly large gorilla. Imogen was a few metres ahead, frowning at it with her face pressed to the wall of the enclosure.

'Africa,' said Mr Stewart. 'But most of them were born at the zoo. Look here – can you read the sign?'

'This one's my favourite,' said Imogen, wrinkling her nose and blowing air into her cheeks in an effort to look like the gorilla. 'Can we take him home?'

'You'll have to ask the zookeeper very nicely,' Mrs Stewart said. 'But shall we have a look at the flamingos first?'

Imogen started to shake her head, and explain that

she would much rather see the wolverines because their name sounded made up, when Mr Stewart barked that everyone should follow *him*, and marched off in the general direction of the lions.

'Why are we going this way?' asked Mrs Stewart. 'Imogen wants to see the flamingos.'

'The *wolverines*!' Imogen corrected. She was staring down at the map, which she had stolen from her mother's handbag, and without looking where she was going trod on the back of Arthur's shoe.

'Well, Arthur wants to see the lions,' said Mr Stewart firmly.

'I'd rather have an ice cream,' said Arthur, glaring at his sister and pulling his shoe back on to his foot. It was the sight of an ice-cream stand that had caused him to stop so suddenly.

'Why do you want an ice cream?' said Imogen. 'It's freezing.'

'Well, perhaps the flamingos would make a good

compromise,' Mrs Stewart suggested.

'That's not a compromise – that's just doing what you want to do,' said Mr Stewart.

'You're only saying that because you want to see the lions!'

Eventually they decided that, provided they were quick, they would have time for everything, but Mr Stewart spent so long looking at the lions, and Imogen spent so long looking at the wolverines, that they ended up with no time left for the flamingos at all.

'Well, that's it!' said Mrs Stewart, in her cross-but-pretending-to-be-polite voice. 'We'll have to go home – the zoo's about to close!'

'But we haven't seen the penguins!' cried Arthur. 'You said we'd see them last!'

'We can have a quick look on our way out,' said Mrs Stewart reluctantly. 'We have to go past them anyway.'

The penguins were outside, with their own beach and a great big pool of water that they were happily diving in and out of. Imogen watched them excitedly and cheered whenever one made a particularly big splash, while Arthur sat a short distance away from her, drawing a picture in his notebook.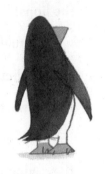

'Imogen, look,' said Arthur suddenly. One of the smallest penguins had walked right up to the glass, and was peering at him.

'Oh, he wants to be our friend!' said Imogen, rushing to join her brother.

'*My* friend,' Arthur corrected.

'Don't be mean,' said Imogen. 'He can be my friend too.'

The penguin tapped its beak against the glass, and looked from Imogen to Arthur and back again.

'Look!' cried Imogen. 'He likes us!'

When they walked along the edge of the enclosure,

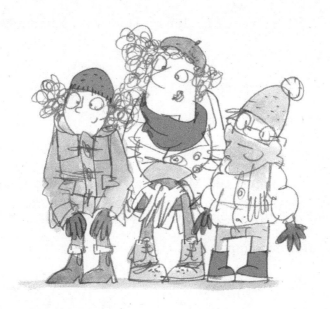

the little penguin waddled beside them, as if it knew exactly what they were thinking, and when they stopped, it stopped too, and squawked and shook its wings.

'I think he's the best penguin here,' said Arthur.

The penguin squawked again, and looked pleased with itself.

'Imogen! Arthur! There you are!' Mrs Stewart appeared suddenly through the crowd. 'What *have* you been doing? It's time to go home.'

'We've made friends with a penguin!' said Imogen. 'Can we keep him? Please?'

Both children were crouching close to the glass, staring at the penguin longingly.

'Please?' said Arthur.

'Come on,' said Mrs Stewart, reaching out a hand for Arthur to hold. 'We can't stay any longer or we'll be late for supper.'

Arthur looked reluctant, so Mrs Stewart gently rolled her eyes and crouched down to face the penguin. 'And *you*, Mr Penguin, must come and stay with us whenever you like. Penguins are always very welcome at our house.'

The penguin looked up at her blankly, and ruffled its feathers.

'There, will that do?' said Mrs Stewart to Imogen and Arthur. 'Can we head home now?'

'All right,' grumbled Arthur, and they followed their mother out towards the gift shop.

CHAPTER TWO

A Penguin Comes to Stay

Back home, the Stewarts settled into one of the early evenings that December tends to demand. The sky had fallen asleep with even more enthusiasm than it had done the day before, and no one was left with any choice but to eat crumpets with butter by the fireside, and wait for supper to finish cooking.

Mr and Mrs Stewart sat on the sofa, watching the news, while the children crouched by the coffee table, squabbling over a jigsaw puzzle.

'Keep your voice down, Arthur,' said Mr Stewart. 'I can't hear the telly.'

'Imogen's hidden a piece of puzzle,' said Arthur sulkily.

'I have not!' said Imogen. 'Arthur hid it!'

Mr Stewart sighed and went to check on the lasagne. 'It looks like it might snow soon,' he said when he came back.

'Really?' said Imogen. 'How can you tell?'

The windows of the living room were foggy with condensation, and Imogen rushed over to wipe one clean with the back of her hand, and stare into the darkness. Outside it was foggy, and the Christmas lights of the corner shop opposite gave the misty air a tinge of yellow. She couldn't see any snow, but it did look cold – as much as outside *can* look cold when one is busy being warm by the fire.

'I think there's someone by the lamp post,' said Imogen suddenly.

'They're probably just walking past,' Mrs Stewart said.

'No,' said Imogen. 'They've stopped.' Then, after a moment, she added, 'They're very small.'

'Well, come away from the window,' said Mr Stewart. 'I'm sure no one wants you staring at them.'

Imogen went to help her brother with the puzzle again. Then, about a minute later, the doorbell rang.

'Supper's nearly ready!' Mr Stewart grumbled. 'Who goes ringing around at this time?' He stood up reluctantly from the sofa, and went to answer the door.

'Erm, Rachel . . .' Mr Stewart's voice sounded nervously from the hallway a few moments later.

'Yes, dear?' Mrs Stewart called.

'I was just wondering, Rachel, why there's a penguin at the door.'

'A *penguin*?' said Mrs Stewart.

The children looked up from their jigsaw, looked

at each other and then raced into the hallway. Their mother quickly followed.

It was true: there was a penguin at the door.

In fact, it was the very same penguin the children

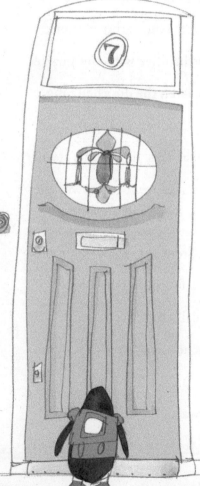

had seen at the zoo just a few hours earlier. And now it was waiting on the doorstep, with a small orange rucksack and a patient expression on its face.

'You haven't accidentally ordered anything online, have you?' Mr Stewart asked.

'What – a penguin?' said Mrs Stewart.

'Well, there was that mix-up last week with the teabags—'

'Yes, James, but a *penguin*?'

Mr Stewart frowned. 'No,' he said. 'I suppose that *would* be rather difficult, wouldn't it?'

The penguin looked at them blankly.

Arthur coughed, and tapped his mother on the arm. 'You did say, Mummy, that he could come to stay whenever he liked.'

Mrs Stewart looked alarmed. 'Why, yes, I suppose I *did* say that – but I didn't really mean . . .'

'You should never say things you don't mean!' Imogen piped up.

Mr and Mrs Stewart looked at each other.

'What are we going to do?' asked Mrs Stewart.

'Well, I suppose –' said Mr Stewart slowly – 'I suppose, given that he's knocked on the door, that we ought to invite him in for supper.'

'Yes,' Mrs Stewart nodded. 'That makes a lot of sense.'

'Can we keep him?' cried Imogen.

'We'll take him back to the zoo in the morning,' Mrs

Stewart corrected. 'He's obviously lost.' She turned to the penguin, and looked down at it kindly. 'Well then, Mr Penguin, I suppose you'd better come in and have something to eat.'

But the penguin had already waddled into the hall. Mr Stewart shut the door behind it, and politely took its bag.

'Do penguins like lasagne?' Arthur wondered aloud as they all went through to the kitchen.

It turned out that this penguin liked lasagne a lot. Its table manners, however, left much to be desired. The penguin, who sat at the head of the table, had finished

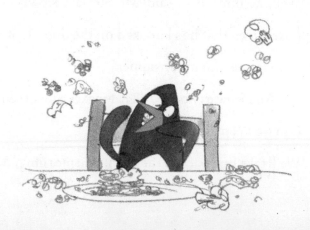

almost all of its lasagne before anyone else had started eating, splattered half of it on to the floor, and never once bothered with a knife and fork.

Meanwhile Gizmo, the cat, took one look at it and shot upstairs to the bathroom to hide in the laundry basket.

'Gosh,' said Mrs Stewart through a nervous laugh. 'Don't they feed you well at the zoo?'

The penguin blinked at her.

Suddenly Imogen pulled her chair close to the table and tried to eat *her* lasagne without a knife and fork too.

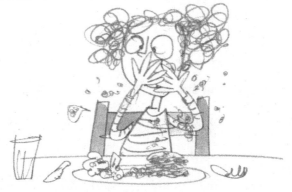

'Imogen!' said Mrs Stewart. 'Stop that!'

'You didn't tell the penguin off,' Imogen retorted.

'The penguin is a *guest*,' said Mrs Stewart. 'And you are *not* a large flightless seabird. Is that clear?'

'Yes, Mum,' said Imogen sulkily, and sat properly again. 'What does it say on his bag, Dad?'

The rucksack was quite old and ragged-looking. At the top, dangling from a strap, was something that looked like a name label.

Mr Stewart put his glasses on and leaned across the table. 'It says Einstein,' he said.

'Einstein?' said Arthur.

'Yes,' said Mr Stewart. 'I suppose that must be what he's called.'

'Well, Einstein,' said Mrs Stewart kindly, 'I hope you enjoyed your supper.'

Einstein looked at her gratefully and shook the feathers on his neck.

'I wonder what's in his bag,' said Imogen.

Mrs Stewart was halfway through a sentence that

sounded an awful lot like, 'It's very rude to look through other people's things,' when Imogen jumped up and undid the zip, tipping the rucksack over as she did so. It burst open.

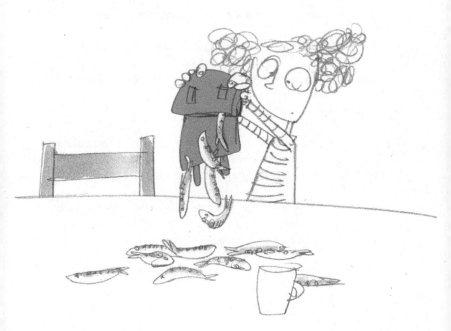

'Oh, gosh!' said Mrs Stewart through another nervous laugh, as several silver fish flopped out on to the dining-room table. 'I suppose that's what penguins eat, isn't it?'

'You certainly came prepared, didn't you?' said Mr Stewart heartily. 'We'd better keep these in the fridge.' He scooped the fish into a bowl and rushed away with them.

'Now,' said Mrs Stewart a few moments later, after the excitement of the fish had died down, 'we should work out where you're going to sleep, Einstein. Children – clear the table, please.'

Imogen and Arthur had never cleared the table so quickly. They had probably never cleared the table so badly, either – but everyone was far too preoccupied with the presence of a penguin to take much notice.

Mr Stewart fetched Arthur's old baby blankets from the airing cupboard, while Mrs Stewart pointed Einstein to the armchair by the fire. He seemed very happy with his own chair to sleep on, and belly-flopped straight on to the cushion while Imogen draped one of the blankets over his back.

'Can we read the bedtime story downstairs with

Einstein?' asked Arthur, and Mrs Stewart looked just about ready to agree when Imogen pointed out that Einstein was already fast asleep, and everyone tiptoed up the stairs to bed.

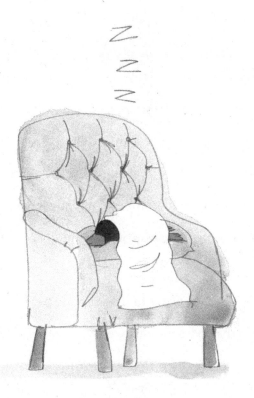

CHAPTER THREE

Sunday Breakfast

Einstein was still asleep when Mrs Stewart crept down the stairs to make coffee early next morning. He was breathing deeply from his chair near the fireplace, so that the air that rushed through his beak sounded like something between a snore and a foghorn, and made Mrs Stewart jump.

'Gosh,' she said to herself shakily, and turned on the television in order to listen to the news.

After that, Mrs Stewart went to boil the kettle in the kitchen, and opened the fridge to reach for the milk.

On this particular morning, however, the milk had been pushed a few centimetres back from its normal place, and Mrs Stewart found herself clutching a small handful of silver fish.

She jumped back, screeching, in response to which Einstein woke up, squawking, and Mr Stewart came barrelling down the stairs, ready to swat something with his newspaper.

'Ah, yes,' said Mr Stewart, pausing when he spotted Einstein, and huffing and puffing several times. 'Penguin,' he said helpfully. 'Just a penguin.'

'I *know*, James,' said Mrs Stewart. 'Why is the fridge full of fish?'

'Well, I had to put them somewhere,' said Mr Stewart defensively. 'And they'd start to smell pretty quickly in the cupboard, you know.'

Mrs Stewart rolled her eyes and carried on making the coffee.

'What's going on?' Imogen's voice piped up, and

her parents turned to see her walking down the stairs in her dressing gown, rubbing her eyes sleepily.

'Oh, nothing,' said her father. 'Just a penguin. We're about to call the zoo.'

Imogen stopped, and her face darkened. 'No, Dad, you can't!'

'What do you mean?' said Mr Stewart, picking up his phone. 'Don't you want him to go home?'

'But he's happy here!' said Imogen.

Everyone turned to the sofa, where Einstein was cheerily belly-flopping after a passing bluebottle.

'Won't he be happier at home, with his penguin parents?'

'What if he ran away on purpose?' said Imogen. 'Maybe they're mean to him at the zoo, and don't give him any lasagne!'

Mr Stewart started to dial the number from the phone book. Imogen watched him, glowered, opened and closed her mouth several times, and then stormed back up the stairs in a whirlwind of pyjamas and slippers.

'Ah, hello,' said Mr Stewart, in his businesslike telephone voice. 'London Zoo? James Stewart speaking. Yes. No. Not a ticket enquiry. No, wait – Look here. We seem to have got hold of one of your penguins.'

There was a long pause.

'Hello?' Mr Stewart continued. 'Yes, of course, do fetch your manager. Yes— Hello? Hi. One of your penguins, yes. We think it must have followed us home from our visit yesterday. Stayed the night, seems happy enough, but perhaps you could send someone to collect it?'

There was another pause.

'Rachel!' said Mr Stewart, aghast. 'They hung up on me!'

'Well, it is a very strange request,' said Mrs Stewart, handing him his coffee. 'Maybe it would help if you explained everything a bit more, and didn't talk so matter-of-factly. Here, let *me* have a go.'

Mrs Stewart took the phone from her husband, and dialled the same number.

'Hello? Now, look, I know this must sound very silly, and the truth is we're just as confused as you are, but the penguin we spoke to at your zoo yesterday has shown up on our doorstep, and as you can imagine we're at a bit of a loss.'

She paused to listen, and took a sip of coffee. 'No? Oh – hang on. But there *is* a penguin here. I—' She pulled the phone away from her ear. 'James, they hung up on me too!'

'Ha!' said Mr Stewart.

'James, this is *not* a competition!'

'Oh, yes,' said Mr Stewart bashfully. 'I suppose not, dear. Sorry.'

'They said they aren't missing any penguins, and that if we prank-call them again they'll report us to the police.'

'Ah,' said Mr Stewart gravely. 'I see.'

Mr and Mrs Stewart sat down at the kitchen table and looked troubled.

'Suppose we *did* keep him?' said Mr Stewart, after a very long pause.

'Don't be ridiculous,' Mrs Stewart snapped.

'No, no, of course not, dear – you're quite right.'

They both turned to the armchair where Einstein, bored at last of the bluebottle, had started to watch the news. The presenter, a short man with a big nose, was talking about the weather in Australia. Einstein squawked vaguely, in a way that suggested he was listening.

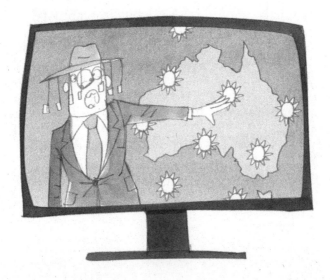

'He does fit in rather well, though, doesn't he?' said Mr Stewart.

Mrs Stewart took a thoughtful sip of coffee. 'Yes,' she said eventually. 'He certainly seems to, but he must be so lonely! Imagine how you'd feel, dear, if you were forced to live among a colony of penguins.'

Mr Stewart's eyes glazed over, as if he was considering the idea, and wasn't entirely opposed to it.

Suddenly a thunder of feet came rattling down the stairs, and Imogen and Arthur rushed into the kitchen.

'You *can't* send him back to the zoo!' said Imogen.

'We've googled it!' said Arthur.

'Animals shouldn't be kept in captivity,' said Imogen, though she stumbled over the last word slightly because it was very long and she was much too cross to remember it properly. 'They should be free to go wherever they want. And Einstein wants to stay here – and it's his right to be allowed to!'

'How do you *know* he wants to stay here, darling?' Mrs Stewart asked.

Einstein squawked from over by the telly.

'*See*,' said Imogen. 'That squawk means "I want to stay here and live with you forever".'

Einstein gave another smaller squawk, and went on watching the news.

Mrs Stewart sighed resignedly. 'Well, the zoo doesn't seem to want him, so I'm afraid he might *have* to stay with us until we work out what to do with him.'

Imogen and Arthur grinned at each other.

'What are those labels on his bag anyway?' Mrs Stewart asked.

Mr Stewart put his reading glasses on and pulled the rucksack over. 'They look like flight labels,' he said.

'Flight labels?' said Mrs Stewart. 'From where?'

Einstein looked up, hopped down from the armchair and waddled over to join them all at the kitchen table.

'This one says Sydney to London.' Mr Stewart frowned. 'How odd – it's only from last week.'

'What have you been doing in Australia, Einstein?' said Imogen.

Einstein stared up at them and tilted his head to one side.

'Maybe he's an Australian penguin,' said Arthur.

'There aren't any penguins in Australia,' said Imogen knowingly. 'It's too hot.'

'There are *some* penguins in Australia,' Mr Stewart corrected. 'On the beaches.'

'But penguins live in Antarctica!'

'Well, he *might* be from Antarctica, but he might be from Australia.'

Einstein gave an excited hoot, and everyone turned to look at him.

'Interesting,' said Mr Stewart, and then repeated himself. 'Antarctica?' he said.

Einstein looked blank.

'Australia?'

Einstein hooted again, and bounced slightly on his little webbed feet.

'He can understand what we're saying,' said Mr Stewart in amazement.

'I knew he did!' said Arthur excitedly. 'You do understand us, don't you?'

Einstein gave Arthur a look as if to suggest that he did.

'What else is in his bag?' said Imogen. 'There might be more clues.' She started to grab hold of it, but stopped herself. 'If you don't mind us looking, of course,' she added politely.

Einstein shrugged his flippers, as if to suggest that he didn't.

Mr Stewart had a look. Now that all the fish were gone, they could see that Einstein had brought several other things with him too – all a little slimy with fish scales. Several photographs were scattered across the

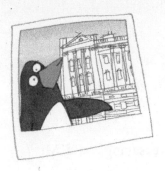

bottom, and a small Polaroid camera sat in the corner, wrapped in a handkerchief.

Einstein squawked loudly from the floor and flapped his flippers impatiently.

Mr Stewart looked a little frightened. 'Oh, dear. What does he want now?' he whispered.

'He just wants to get on the table so he can see,' Arthur explained. He picked Einstein up and placed him on top of one of Mrs Stewart's cookbooks.

Einstein waddled across the table towards his bag. He stuck his head inside and started to pick

the photographs up, one by one, and place them down on the table. The first was of Einstein in Australia, outside the Sydney Opera House.

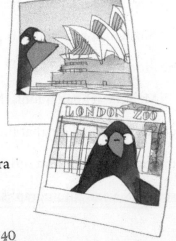

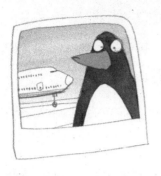 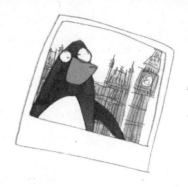

The second was Einstein at an airport, and another showed him arriving in London. The next few were selfies: outside Buckingham Palace and the Houses of Parliament, and hiding in a handbag in the back of a taxi. The most recent one showed Einstein at the zoo.

'Oh . . .' said Mrs Stewart slowly, as if something very important was occurring to her. 'So Einstein isn't from London Zoo after all?'

Einstein gave a resigned squawk, to thank her for finally realising.

'Well, that explains why they didn't take our calls,' said Mrs Stewart. 'But, Einstein, how on *earth* did you get inside the zoo and back out again, without anyone noticing?'

'He's very little,' Imogen pointed out. 'He can probably squeeze into tight spaces.'

Einstein gave a sort of nod – as much of a nod as a very little penguin is able to give – and stepped in and out of Mrs Stewart's handbag by way of demonstration.

Mrs Stewart looked impressed. 'They call you Einstein for a reason, I suppose.'

'What do we do then, Mummy?' said Arthur. 'Can we keep him?'

'Well, I don't know,' said Mrs Stewart. 'I suppose, if he'd *like* to stay with us – and it doesn't seem like he has anywhere to go . . .'

'So we're a hotel for holidaying Australian penguins now?' Mr Stewart scoffed.

'Oh, come on, James,' said Mrs Stewart. 'You were the one who wanted to keep him a minute ago.'

Mr Stewart grumbled his assent: he didn't really mean his scoffs and mutters, but thought that, between himself and Mrs Stewart, one of them always needed to be acting sensibly, even if they both got distracted and had to take it in turns.

'But only until we work out where he comes from,' he said. 'I don't suppose we can pack him off to Australia if he doesn't have a home to go to . . .'

'Well, Einstein,' said Mrs Stewart, 'you've a place to stay with us for as long as you need one. Penguins are always very welcome at our house.'

CHAPTER FOUR

Einstein Goes to School

Imogen got ready more quickly than usual on Monday morning, and came downstairs just in time for breakfast – though she was still brushing her teeth, and appeared to be missing a sock. Mrs Stewart, who was a teacher at the big school, was frantically looking for the homework she'd been marking, while Mr Stewart shook crumbs out of the toaster, and wondered how busy work would be at the hospital.

'Where's your brother?' asked Mr Stewart, as

Imogen yawned and dropped toothpaste down her skirt.

'Dunno,' said Imogen. She spat into the sink and sat down at the table.

'What was that?' asked Mrs Stewart. '*Dunno?*'

Imogen, as a matter of fact, did know: her brother was still in bed. He had fallen asleep with Gizmo the cat on one side of his pillow, and Einstein on the other. Neither creature had seemed particularly pleased with this arrangement, but neither had been willing to give up their turf, and all in all the conflict had made all three of them far too tired to get up when Arthur's alarm clock rang.

'Arthur!' Mr Stewart shouted up the stairs. 'Breakfast! School!'

There were several loud stomping noises, and Arthur appeared in the kitchen two minutes later, shortly followed by the cat, and then by Einstein, who was slower on account of having to hop from step to step.

'Do we really still have to go to school now that we have a penguin?' asked Arthur sleepily.

'Of course,' said Mrs Stewart. 'I'm sure little penguins have to go to school just like little people do.'

'I'm not little,' said Imogen, though this was mostly to herself.

'I don't want to go to school,' said Arthur, lifting Einstein up on to the chair between his own and Imogen's. It was stacked with a pile of books to help bring him up to table-height.

Einstein looked at Arthur and gave a concerned cluck.

'Arthur doesn't like school,' Imogen explained. 'He's only just started, and he doesn't have any friends yet.'

'*Imogen*,' Mrs Stewart scolded. 'Don't talk about your brother like that!'

'Sorry,' said Imogen. 'I didn't mean it in a bad way!'

Arthur rubbed his eyes groggily and started to

butter his toast, while Mrs Stewart flitted round the kitchen, trying to work out what penguins liked for breakfast.

'Just give him some more herring, Rachel,' said Mr Stewart tiredly.

'But he had that for supper *last* night!' Mrs Stewart sighed. 'Won't he get bored of eating the same thing?'

'He's a penguin, not a food critic,' said Mr Stewart. 'Put some chocolate spread on them if you think he wants garnish.'

Mrs Stewart sighed again, but went along with the idea. 'Imogen!' she cried, as she put Einstein's breakfast plate down in front of him. '*Try* not to get butter on the penguin!'

'I didn't mean to – I slipped!' said Imogen, who was now trying to scoop the butter off Einstein's head with her spoon, and put it back into the tub. Einstein didn't seem to notice, or care. He was too busy gobbling down the silver fish.

'Well, he seems to like the herrings!' said Mrs Stewart, who spotted the spoon and intercepted it before darting over to the kettle to make coffee.

'I'm not surprised, dear,' said Mr Stewart. 'He's a penguin.'

'Well, you know,' said Mrs Stewart vaguely. 'I'm sure they all have different tastes, and that sort of thing.'

Mr Stewart stopped chewing his toast for a moment, and turned to Arthur, frowning. 'Hang on, did that penguin sleep in your room last night?'

Arthur nodded. 'I was reading him a bedtime story.'

'You can't read,' said Imogen.

'Yes I can!' said Arthur.

'Is that hygienic?' asked Mr Stewart.

Mrs Stewart shrugged. 'Einstein seems clean enough,' she said, which, given the butter and the chocolate and the herrings, was no longer strictly true. 'And the cat sleeps where he likes, doesn't he?'

'Einstein will sleep downstairs tomorrow,' said Mr Stewart decidedly. 'Bedtime stories can be done in the sitting room.'

'What about while we're at school and you're at work?' asked Imogen.

'Can he come to school with us?' asked Arthur.

Mr Stewart frowned. He'd forgotten to think about that.

'Einstein will have to stay at home,' he said eventually. 'We'll leave some water in the bathtub, and put some herrings out on the table. Now, let's sort it out quickly because we're *all* running late.'

The usual leaving-the-house rush ensued. Imogen's second sock was retrieved from the larder, Gizmo was rescued from the laundry basket, and Einstein was given a pat on the head and left in the kitchen.

'Bye, Einstein!' said Imogen sadly as Mrs Stewart frantically tried to brush her hair into a ponytail. 'We'll be back again later!'

'I'll drive you to school,' said Mr Stewart, checking his watch as everybody rushed outside. 'You've run out of time to catch the bus. Car! Now!'

Everyone jumped in. The doors slammed shut and the car started to pull out of the driveway. Then,

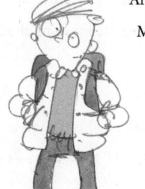

'Arthur! Where's Arthur?' cried Mrs Stewart.

'I'm here,' said Arthur, suddenly appearing on the gravel beside the car, and slinging his bag over his shoulder. He opened the door and hopped in.

'Where did you go?' said Mr Stewart, narrowing his eyes.

'I left something in the kitchen.' Arthur gave an innocent little smile and adjusted the zips on his backpack.

Mr Stewart shrugged and started to drive.

*

When Arthur walked into the classroom for maths that morning, he felt twice as tall as usual. He chose a table in the middle of the room and tucked his backpack carefully between his feet. Then, as he waited for class to start, he leaned down and undid the zip slightly. Two shiny grey eyes blinked happily up at him.

'Make sure you keep quiet,' whispered Arthur. 'And stay in the bag, okay?'

The first half of the lesson went smoothly. Einstein didn't make a peep, aside from one small snore somewhere in the middle of the three times table; but as soon as Mr Smith started testing the class he woke up, and gave a sharp wriggle.

'Shh,' Arthur whispered. 'I know it's boring, but there's only ten minutes left.' He said it so quietly, however, that he wasn't sure Einstein could hear him.

'What's two times four?' Mr Smith asked, eyeing Arthur severely.

Arthur looked up from his backpack, and stared blankly at the whiteboard. 'Uh,' he said. 'Ten.' Einstein gave a lurch, and pecked him repeatedly on the ankle. 'I mean eight.'

'Good. So what's eight divided by two?'

Jack Jones, the boy who sat on Arthur's right, started to snigger.

Arthur felt his neck go hot. He didn't like being asked questions in front of the class, and Einstein was making it worse by moving about. Arthur couldn't think properly, and was just about to confess that he didn't know the answer when Einstein gave him four more pecks on the ankle.

Arthur paused, frowning. 'Four?' he guessed at last.

'Yes, exactly,' said Mr Smith, looking surprised. He turned to Arthur's neighbour. 'Layla, what's two times five?'

Arthur looked down at Einstein, who was staring up at him from inside the bag. 'Can you do maths?' he whispered incredulously.

Einstein ruffled his feathers smugly.

'Take your homework from the pile as you leave the room!' Mr Smith announced a few minutes later as the bell rang and the class started to file out of the room and in the direction of the playground. He looked down suspiciously as Arthur ducked past. 'And remember, everyone, homework should be your own work.'

Einstein soon settled down into the school routine.

Gizmo had almost always eaten Einstein's herrings by the time the Stewarts got home and, if Arthur ran upstairs quickly enough, he could leave Einstein splashing innocently around in the bathtub for somebody else to discover.

In fact, after just a few days, Arthur found it

difficult to remember what *not* having a penguin in his backpack used to feel like. It was comforting carrying Einstein around with his books and pencils. He kept the backpack unzipped slightly. When his family was looking the other way, Einstein could poke his head out and admire all the parts of London he hadn't seen before, and surprise old ladies on the bus. And, whenever Einstein had to keep his head *in*side the backpack, Arthur could walk around, knowing he had a secret, and it made him feel important.

Although maths was boring, the scariest part of the day, in Arthur's opinion, was lunch. Lucinda the dinner lady never seemed to smile, and she made Arthur feel as if he had done something very wrong just by coming to get food from her. He hated the sloppiness of the overcooked vegetables, and the fact that he couldn't leave the table without eating them. And, scariest of all, he never knew where to sit. Sometimes Imogen would let Arthur sit with *her* friends, but there wasn't always room, and she wasn't always eating at the same time as him. She preferred not to have her brother following her around anyway – not now that she was nine.

On the first Friday lunchtime since Einstein had moved in, Arthur took his fishfingers and chips from Lucinda, stammered a thank you and went to sit at a big table by himself, where he could pass chips to Einstein without anyone noticing, and stare at the cars going past outside the window. No one took backpacks into the lunch hall, so Arthur had transferred Einstein into his jacket in the secrecy of the changing room.

He had been feeding Einstein chips quite happily for several minutes when a voice took him by surprise. Arthur dropped the chip he was holding on to his plate and quickly shook his jacket, to warn Einstein to keep still.

The voice belonged to Theo, a new boy in Arthur's class who had lots of wavy black hair. 'Hello,' said Theo a second time, and sat down. 'You're Arthur, aren't you?'

Arthur nodded through a mouthful of squishy broccoli.

'I'm Theo,' said Theo.

'I know,' said Arthur, swallowing. 'You're in my class.'

'Yeah,' Theo grinned. 'You're the one who's good at maths!'

Einstein wriggled again, and Arthur's ears went pink. He had finished his food now, but Theo, beside him, was only just tucking into a great big fishfinger. Arthur buttoned up his jacket and hissed at Einstein to be quiet.

'What was that?' said Theo.

'Nothing,' said Arthur.

'Did you say "be quiet"?'

'No,' said Arthur. 'I said thank you.'

'Oh,' said Theo, through a mouthful of fish. 'That's okay.'

Arthur glanced down. Einstein had stopped moving, but his orange beak was poking out from the jacket as he eyed Theo's lunch.

'Einstein, *no*,' Arthur whispered sternly.

But it was too late. In a flurry of flippers, Einstein leaped out of Arthur's jacket, grabbed a fishfinger right off Theo's plate and disappeared with it under the table.

'Einstein!' shouted Arthur.

'What was *that*?' Theo leaped up in surprise and sent his plate and cutlery flying.

Imogen, who was just a few tables away, stared at them with wide eyes.

'*What is going on over there?*' Lucinda the dinner lady's voice echoed across the room. She came marching over, fish slice in hand, and glowered menacingly.

Arthur gulped. Einstein was still under the table, eating Theo's fish as if nothing was the matter. No one else seemed to have noticed him yet – no one except Theo and Imogen – but it wouldn't be long before they did.

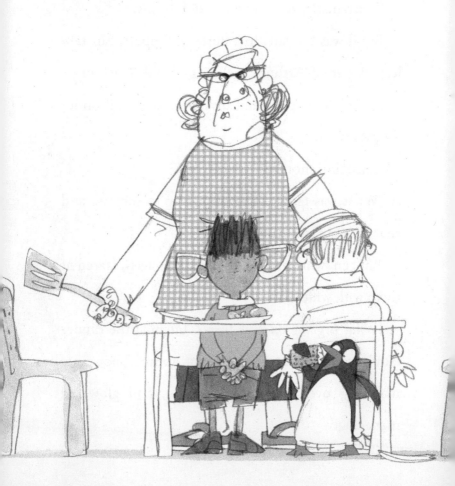

'It was my fault!' said Theo suddenly.

Arthur stared at him.

'I don't like loud noises in my dining room,' said Lucinda loudly.

'I'm sorry,' said Theo. 'Arthur told me a very funny joke, which is why I shouted. And then I dropped my plate.' As he was talking, Theo nudged his jacket off his chair and on to the top of Einstein's head. It was a big jacket, and it covered Einstein neatly.

Lucinda narrowed her eyes. 'Jokes,' she said slowly, 'should be told *quietly*, if at all.'

'Sorry,' said Theo a second time. 'It won't happen again.'

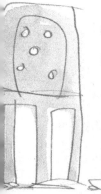

Lucinda scowled again, as if she knew something was amiss, but couldn't tell what. She retreated reluctantly to her kitchen.

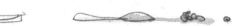

With Lucinda a safe distance away, Theo crouched down and scooped up Einstein, bundling him up inside the jacket, and turned to look at Arthur. The two boys grinned at each other and hurried out of the dining room.

Arthur and Theo ran as fast as they could to the end of the playground, where they couldn't be seen from the school. Theo placed his jacket down on the ground and Einstein came tumbling out of it, his beak still full of fishfinger. He hopped up and shook his flippers for balance.

'You have a penguin!' said Theo at last.

'His name's Einstein,' said Arthur. 'Thanks for covering for us.'

'Where did you find him?'

Arthur hesitated for a moment. 'At the zoo,' he said. 'He followed us home.'

'That's the coolest thing I've ever heard!' said Theo.

'He's been in my backpack all week, actually,' said Arthur. Then, panicking for a moment, he added, 'Do you promise not to tell anyone?'

'It's okay,' said Theo. 'I won't.'

He spat on his hand and held it out for Arthur to shake, and Arthur – a little confused because he'd never seen anyone do that before – did the same.

Just then Imogen appeared outside the dining hall and came marching across the playground towards them.

'Uh-oh,' said Arthur under his breath.

'What?'

'It's my sister. Hide the penguin again.'

'So you've been taking Einstein to school, have you?' said Imogen, as soon as she was within earshot. She raised an eyebrow and crossed her arms, just like their mother did when she was cross.

'No,' said Arthur.

'Yes you have.'

'How do you know?'

'Because his foot is poking out from underneath your friend's jacket.'

Theo looked embarrassed and tried to nudge the jacket over the stray foot.

'Well, I've seen him now,' said Imogen, 'so you might as well admit it.'

'Don't tell Dad,' Arthur pleaded.

Imogen pursed her lips and thought for a moment. 'Okay, but I want shotgun in the car for the next month,' she said.

'What? You can't do that!'

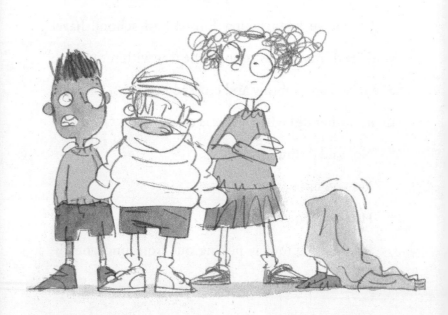

'So I can tell Mum and Dad?'

'Okay,' said Arthur. '*Fine.*'

'See you at home time!' said Imogen sweetly, and she disappeared back across the playground.

CHAPTER FIVE

A New Friend and a Lost One

The weekend was snowy.

It was a bright, bossy sort of snow, with great big flakes that fell slowly and softly like the sky really meant them. The sort of light, white winter's day when noises are muffled and London seems ready to burst with happiness at simply being awake.

Breakfast had occurred without incident, snowballs had been born off the window ledges, and Imogen was curled up on her favourite cushion, with a pile of detective books and a telescope. She had read most of these books already, but she'd never much liked the idea of carrying *one* book around without any of its friends, or of having *one* thing kept neatly when she could have a great big messy pile of stuff instead.

The current book was a mystery about a stolen painting, and Imogen was enjoying it very much. The main character was a detective called Inspector Bucket, who was very clever, and always found clues in the places you'd least expect them. At the end of each page she would turn to the window to check that it was still snowing, or look through the telescope to see if it made the flakes look bigger – it mostly just made them look blurry.

Arthur was playing outside with his new friend, and Imogen wasn't sure how she felt about it. She had played with them too, for a bit, but usually when she played with Arthur she could make the rules. Now that Theo had joined in, they were throwing the snowballs too hard, and hadn't been interested in making snow angels. And so Imogen had decided all at once that, being nine, she was much too grown up for both brothers *and* snow, and had come inside to hide in the house.

Imogen's favourite cushion was in the upstairs corridor, next to a round window that looked out over the garden, where the boys were cheering as Einstein slid around on his belly. Imogen watched them through her telescope.

Then, remembering that she wasn't interested in that sort of thing, she pointed the telescope upwards and examined the roofs on the houses across the street instead. When she looked back down a moment later, the boys were over by the garden wall, and Einstein had disappeared.

A sudden bouncing of feet up the stairs seemed to answer her confusion, and she turned to see Einstein waddling down the corridor towards her.

Imogen, pleased as she was to see him, looked at

Einstein suspiciously. She'd been feeling a little hard done by: Arthur had seen Einstein first, and Arthur had taken him to school, and Arthur had been able to introduce him to his friends, and Einstein probably preferred Arthur too. Imogen's friends didn't know about Einstein – and how could she tell them if Einstein was never hidden in her backpack to prove it?

Einstein looked at her sincerely and stretched his flippers out, like he did before a particularly large squawk.

Imogen smiled despite herself. 'Hello, Einstein,' she said.

Einstein looked visibly relieved, and gave a smaller, softer squawk, as if to ask her how she was.

'I'm reading books about detectives,' said Imogen. 'Some of them have very long words, but I can understand them anyway.'

He tilted his head to one side, the way he did when he didn't understand something.

'Detectives are people who solve mysteries,' Imogen explained. 'They use clues to look for lost things.'

Einstein seemed interested in this, so she handed him one of the books.

'Here,' she said. 'Have a look.'

He leaned over and peered down his beak at the front cover. Then he turned the book over with his foot, and read the back.

'That's one of my favourites,' said Imogen. 'It's about a kidnapping. Oh – a kidnapping is when baddies steal someone away, and ask for lots of money to return them.'

Einstein looked up at her and his little eyes widened.

'But don't worry!' said Imogen. 'Inspector Bucket always gets them back.'

Einstein gave a terrified honk, and then waddle-ran as fast as he could back along the corridor and down the stairs. Imogen watched him go. 'Silly penguin,' she said to herself, and carried on reading.

Einstein made a point of sitting next to Imogen at lunch. He waddled up to the chair beside her and bossily squawked to be lifted up.

'We should get him a high chair, really,' said Mrs Stewart.

'*That* implies you think he's staying here forever,' said Mr Stewart tetchily as he balanced Einstein on his usual pile of books.

'You wanted him to stay forever first!' said Mrs Stewart. 'And I'm sorry you're so cross, but I've told you your work trousers will dry-clean.'

'We can't afford to dry-clean our clothes every day for*ever*, Rachel,' Mr Stewart grumbled.

'And we won't! He's making very good progress with his toilet training!'

'He *can* hear you, you know!' cried Imogen

defensively. She turned to look at Einstein and noticed he was holding a piece of paper in his beak, which he placed on the table in front of her.

'He's never *once* made a mess while the children have been at school, has he?' Mrs Stewart went on vaguely.

Imogen picked the paper up to inspect it.

'What did he just give you?' asked Arthur, who had, until that moment, been busily talking to Theo about superheroes.

'It's just another of Einstein's photos of himself,' said Imogen.

Einstein gave an urgent little caw.

'What?' she asked him. 'Isn't it you?' She looked back at the photograph and noticed the little strands of yellow feathers splaying out from the penguin's eyebrows, as well as its reddish eyes, which differed from Einstein's dark ones. 'Oh,' she said. 'It's *not* you.' She turned the photograph over and saw that the

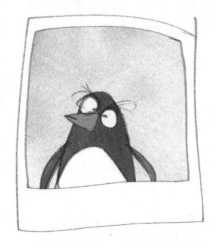

name ISAAC was
written rather messily
on the bottom corner.

'Soup's ready!' Mr
Stewart cried. 'Put that
away, Imogen.'

Imogen shoved the
photograph into her pocket and gave Einstein a quick
little smile, to show him that she wouldn't forget
about it.

'I don't like soup,' whinged Arthur. 'We *al*ways
have soup.'

'You can learn to like soup,' said Mr Stewart, placing
one bowl down in front of him, and another in front
of Theo.

'Einstein doesn't like soup, either,' Imogen pointed
out. 'It gets in his eyes when he tries to drink it.'

'Oh, yes . . .' said Mrs Stewart. 'Do you think he'd
prefer a Pot Noodle?'

'Hey!' said Arthur. '*That*'s not fair!'

'Just give him another raw herring,' said Mr Stewart tiredly. 'And, Arthur, if you complain about my cooking again, then you can have a raw herring too.'

Theo almost spilled his soup from giggling.

Einstein followed Imogen around all afternoon. He stayed beside her for the whole of their walk on the heath, and watched her while she fidgeted over her science homework, and hardly noticed when the boys tried to convince him to play catch with them.

Imogen was both confused and flattered. She didn't smell of herrings or sardines – she even sniffed herself to check – and she looked just the same as usual.

'Why is Einstein staring at you?' said Arthur. He and Theo had come back inside, disappointed by Einstein's disinterest in their games.

'I don't know.' Imogen shrugged. 'He's been doing

it ever since he gave me that photo at lunch.'

Einstein squawked at her, so Imogen took the photo back out of her pocket and looked at it.

'Did you see him before lunch?' asked Theo. 'He disappeared.'

'Yes, he came upstairs to look at my detective books.'

Imogen frowned: it was the mention of detectives and kidnappings that had made Einstein start acting strangely. 'I think the penguin in the photo must be a friend of his or something. He's called Isaac.'

'How do you know his name?' asked Arthur, peering at the photo. 'Isaac,' he read. 'Einstein, did you write that?'

Einstein blinked and nodded.

'Cool!' said Arthur. 'I bet no one else has a penguin who can write!'

Then Theo leaned over Imogen's shoulder and had a look at the photo. 'I like his yellow eyebrows,' he said. 'Where's your friend now, Einstein?'

Einstein squawked again, and shrugged his flippers.

'You don't know?' said Arthur.

Imogen's eyes widened, and suddenly everything fell into place. 'That's right!' she cried. 'His friend must be missing! That's why he was scared when I mentioned kidnappings!'

Einstein quickly nodded his head.

'Perhaps he's been kidnapped and held for ransom by pirates!' she went on excitedly, prompting another scared honk from Einstein. 'Sorry, Einstein – I didn't really mean that . . . But don't worry! We'll get Isaac back.'

Einstein nudged one of Imogen's books towards her, and poked the name on the front cover with his beak.

'Oh, no – Inspector Bucket isn't a real detective,' she explained.

Einstein hung his flippers in disappointment.

'But *I'll* help you!' said Imogen. She tried to speak in a way that was both determined and comforting, just like Inspector Bucket did in her books. 'Arthur, you can be my assistant. Fetch my notebook and magnifying glass!'

'I don't know where they are,' said Arthur. 'Your room's always too messy to find anything.'

'Have you looked at all his other photos?' asked Theo helpfully.

'I think so,' said Imogen, going a little pink at her overenthusiasm, but she agreed that they ought to check.

Theo picked up Einstein's backpack from where it was lying on the floor and started rooting through the pockets.

'We've already seen all of those,' said Arthur, leaning over Theo's shoulder.

Then Theo pulled a different photo out of a different pocket, and turned it over. 'What about this one?'

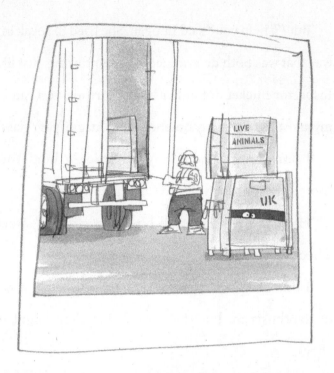

The new photo showed a pile of wooden crates
sitting beside a lorry. One of them had two little
holes in the side, and peering through the holes – just
visible between the shadows – was a pair of eyes. Eyes
surrounded by feathery yellow eyebrows. The box
was labelled in black paint: *UK*.

Imogen gasped, and Arthur grabbed the photo out
of Theo's hand.

'UK?' he read aloud.

'United Kingdom,' Imogen explained. Then she tried to grab the photo from Arthur.

'I know what UK means,' said Arthur crossly, though in actual fact he had been a little too excited to remember. He pushed his sister's hand away. 'It doesn't say where in the UK, though. His friend could be anywhere! Do you think someone kidnapped him from the beach in Australia?'

'Give it here!' said Imogen, leaping at him.

'Stop it!' cried Theo. 'Look at Einstein! You're upsetting him.'

Imogen and Arthur stopped bickering and turned round. Einstein had ruffled up his feathers and was staring down at the surface of the table, hunching his back sadly.

'Now look what you've done!' said Imogen. 'He's upset!'

'It wasn't *my* fault!' said Arthur.

'It's okay, Einstein,' said Imogen. She leaned down and looked him carefully in the eye. 'We're going to help you find him,' she said. 'We promise.'

CHAPTER SIX

Detectives at Work

The woman in the café held the poster at arm's length and frowned at it through her reading glasses. 'Do you have an adult with you?' she asked, looking down at Arthur over the countertop. 'You need an adult with you if you want to put a poster on the noticeboard.'

'He's only six,' said Imogen, stepping away from the cupcakes she had been admiring in the window and putting a hand on her brother's arm. 'But I'll be ten in March. Does that count?'

The waitress glanced at the messy-haired girl in the red duffel coat, and was just about to say something clever when she spotted the penguin poking out of her right-hand pocket. 'But – but—' She shook the poster at them frantically. 'Your penguin's right there,' she squeaked, pointing at Imogen's coat.

Imogen took the poster back from the waitress and placed it down on the counter, so that Arthur's crayon rendition of Isaac's yellow eyebrows stared alarmingly up at the café ceiling. 'It's a *different* penguin,' said Imogen, pointing out the colours, and then running her finger along her own handwriting for emphasis:

Missing Pengwin, Possibly Kid-Napped, Informashion To Be Rewarded.

'See?' she added politely. 'The penguin *we* want is missing, but *this* penguin isn't missing at all!'

The waitress shook her head in disbelief. The café didn't have any rules about penguins. No cats, no dogs, no political leaflets on the noticeboard – but penguins? 'All right, fine,' she said tiredly. 'I'll put it up. Can I take a name, in case anyone responds?'

'DCI Imogen Stewart,' said Imogen. 'And this is my assistant, Arthur.'

'Thank you for your help,' said Arthur, his ears going pink.

'See you again soon,' said Imogen, and then she paused. 'Actually, can we have three of those cupcakes too, please?' She scooped some change out of her pocket and fumbled around with it on the counter. 'One pound, nearly two . . .' she mumbled, as the waitress waited and watched Einstein nervously. 'I think I've got some more change in my other pocket. Is it all right if I take my penguin out so I can have a look?'

'You know what? Have the third cupcake for free,'

said the waitress, placing them down on the counter. 'I'm sure you have lots more posters to hand out, and I wouldn't want to hold you up.'

'Thank you!' said Imogen, beaming, and she took the cupcakes and followed her brother out on to the street.

They sat on the bench outside to eat their cupcakes. Einstein's cupcake was too big for him to eat in one go, so Imogen broke it up into little pieces and threw them into the air for him to catch. Several passers-by stopped and stared, and once or twice some pigeons got in the way – but Einstein would chase them until they flew up on to the café awning to watch from above instead.

'Well done, Einstein!' cried Imogen, clapping, as he grabbed a piece of icing that was about to land in front of another particularly fat pigeon. Yesterday's snow was still on the ground around them, going grey in slushy heaps at the edge of the road. Imogen kicked it about with her boots as they walked off.

'Shall we put a poster up in the bus stop?' asked Arthur.

'Good idea,' said Imogen. She turned round to see Einstein on the verge of a fight with another pigeon, so handed her brother the posters before running over to rescue him. 'Stop it, Einstein,' she scolded, and put him back into her pocket. 'That one's bigger than you!'

Einstein squawked sulkily, and glared at the pigeon from the safety of the duffel coat as it swaggered away down the road.

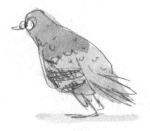

They taped the posters up and down all the parts of town they knew, and kept going until they had run out of posters entirely. Some went in shops, others on signposts, and the biggest was saved for the noticeboard outside the library. Imogen felt particularly proud as she pinned this one up because it was so big, and colourful, and it had her neatest handwriting on it. The name 'Isaac' had been written by Einstein, with a pencil held uncertainly in his beak. Then Imogen had gone over it more neatly with a pen.

She took her detective notebook out of her pocket and put a big tick next to where she had written Missing Pengwin Posters. ✔

The snow restarted as they walked home, coughed down in little spatters by a greying sky and then gathering speed. Big flakes were soon sticking in Imogen's hair and falling down inside Arthur's collar. Einstein nestled further into Imogen's coat pocket and hid his head from sight.

'Do you think we'll find Isaac?' said Arthur.

'Of course!' said Imogen confidently, because she was the oldest. But she was starting to feel less confident with every step. Pinning the posters up had felt like *doing* something. She hadn't thought about what might happen *after* it was done: anything could, or maybe nothing would.

'Before Christmas?' said Arthur.

Einstein poked his head back out of Imogen's pocket for a moment, and blinked at her.

Imogen frowned. Christmas wasn't far away now: there was only a week left of school, and then only a few days of holiday before the day itself. And they couldn't search for Isaac while they were busy at school, could they? They'd be in lessons. They could ask their parents for help – but Mr Stewart often got cross enough about having just *one* penguin about the house. He'd never let Isaac stay too, even if they could find him. And then maybe Einstein wouldn't want to live with them any more.

'Before Christmas,' Imogen agreed. 'I'm absolutely sure of it.'

Mr Stewart narrowed his eyes as the children entered the kitchen. 'Where have you two been?'

'We were playing in the garden,' said Arthur.

'For a whole hour?' said Mr Stewart. 'Together? Without arguing?'

'And we bought cupcakes from the café,' said Imogen.

'You shouldn't leave the garden by yourselves,' said Mrs Stewart, glancing up from her pile of marking.

'It's only across the road!' said Imogen.

'Don't argue with your mother.'

'Sorry,' Imogen mumbled. She took her coat off and placed Einstein down on the floor, where he gave a satisfied chunter and shook the few snowflakes that had lodged themselves in his feathers in a shower down on to the carpet.

Mr Stewart smiled despite himself.

'Where's all my paper gone?' said Mrs Stewart.

'No idea,' said Mr Stewart, turning back to his laptop. 'Never saw it.'

'I had a great big pile of paper right next to the printer! Just this morning!'

The children looked at each other and sidled up the stairs into Arthur's bedroom.

Imogen paced up and down beside Arthur's bed. She scratched her head and tried putting her hands behind her back, and then inside her pockets, and then behind her back again.

'Come on, *think*!' she said, to no one in particular.

'I don't know what I'm supposed to be thinking about,' said Arthur, who was sitting on a beanbag with Einstein, sticking Lego pieces together into a tower.

Imogen didn't know, either, but she wasn't going to let on. 'This is important,' she insisted. 'Einstein needs to find his friend. It's why he's here!'

'Is it?' said Arthur.

Einstein gave a small squawk of agreement.

'I thought you were here because you liked us,' said Arthur, sounding crestfallen.

'He *does* like you, Arthur,' said Imogen. 'But we like him too. And we promised that we'd find his friend. And people who like each other keep their promises. Where's my magnifying glass?'

Arthur picked the magnifying glass up from underneath a cushion and handed it to his sister, who started closely examining Isaac's photograph for the eleventh time that day. She had glued the photo into the first page of her notebook and added lots of arrows around its edges. They formed a spider diagram like the ones she had seen the police do on TV, all leading to lots of important notes: things like:

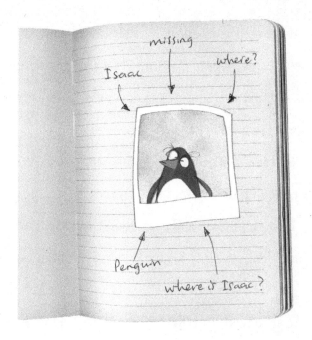

Arthur took his own photo out of his pocket, and looked at it again. It turned out Einstein had had several photos of Isaac – enough for Arthur and Imogen to borrow one each. Still, Arthur wasn't sure what staring at a photo all day could do: it wasn't like they ever changed shape or told you anything different. He put it back into his pocket and went on playing with his Lego.

'I've got the facts, but they just don't add together,'

said Imogen mysteriously. She turned to look out of the window, where the snow had stopped falling and the sky had settled down to darkness. 'Interesting,' she mumbled to herself.

Suddenly Mr Stewart opened the door. 'What are you kids up to?' he said.

Imogen jumped and spun round, quickly tucking her magnifying glass into her back pocket. 'Nothing,' she said.

Mr Stewart turned to the sofa and looked at Arthur, who shrugged, and then at Einstein, who looked blank and tripped over a pillow.

'I know you're up to something,' he said. 'I've never seen you go this long without fighting.'

'It's Einstein,' said Imogen, smiling sweetly. 'He brings us together.'

They all turned to look at the little penguin, who was now face down on the sofa, struggling to push himself up with his flippers. Arthur quickly lifted him on to his feet.

'Hmm,' said Mr Stewart. 'All right. Supper's in ten minutes, so wash your hands . . . and wash that penguin's flippers while you're at it too.'

Imogen felt worse again during supper. Mr Stewart had made her favourite roast chicken, but it was going down all wrong, and her stomach was doing guilty somersaults every time she looked over at Einstein happily eating his herrings. What if she *never* found Isaac? Maybe she had got too far ahead of herself with all those detective promises. She would break Einstein's heart. What could a nine-year-old do to change anything, after all? Maybe Isaac *had* been kidnapped and held for ransom by pirates, and even if Imogen managed to work out what ship he was on she was much too small to beat anyone in a sword fight, and would probably be kidnapped and held for ransom herself. And then who would rescue *her*? She wasn't a detective, she was just a silly little—

'Imogen?' said Mrs Stewart kindly.

'Huh, what?' said Imogen, through a mouthful of potato.

'I was just asking how you'd got on with your science homework? You're miles away!'

'Oh,' said Imogen. 'Yeah. It was easy.'

'Jolly good,' said Mrs Stewart, and turned to Einstein. 'Would you like some gravy with your herrings, dear?'

Mr Stewart rolled his eyes gently. 'What are you thinking about, hmm?' he asked Imogen.

She caught her brother's eye across the table. 'Nothing,' she said quickly.

'You look worried.'

'Oh – I was just thinking about school tomorrow. We have a spelling test.'

'You're good at spelling, aren't you?'

'I'm okay,' said Imogen, stirring a piece of broccoli round her plate with her fork. 'Science is easier.'

'Well! Only a week to go – and then it's the Christmas holidays!'

Imogen smiled.

'Can Einstein stay for Christmas?' asked Arthur.

'Of course!' said Mrs Stewart.

'Well –' Mr Stewart coughed – 'I think we should all remember that Einstein's stay is still on a temporary, take-each-day-as-it-comes basis, just until we work out where he actually lives . . .'

His sentence trailed off: Einstein was blinking at Mr Stewart from the other side of the table, over the top of the white napkin that Mrs Stewart had fixed round his neck for herring spillages.

'But, you know,' Mr Stewart went on vaguely, 'if Christmas comes along and it suits everyone for Einstein to be here, then, well, there's no *specific* reason why not.'

'*Yes!*' Arthur whispered to himself, and Einstein gave a small herring-breathed squawk.

'Can he have his own stocking?' Arthur went on. 'Do you think he'll like Christmas pudding?'

'And *on that note!*' Mr Stewart interrupted. 'It is a school night, and you both need to get ready for bed.'

Imogen looked out of the bathroom window while she brushed her teeth.

The pavement outside was only dimly lit, shadowy beneath the glow that fell from the windows. When she pressed her face against the glass, it felt cold, and little white shadows of fog appeared. She wiped them away with the sleeve of her dressing gown.

Their first poster was dangling forlornly from a battered old lamp post, where the Stewarts' street met the corner of the next street along. Imogen frowned at it. It didn't seem like much use all of a sudden.

Then, just as she was about to turn to spit into the basin, she saw somebody approach it. Imogen gasped despite herself and nearly swallowed her toothpaste.

She couldn't see the somebody's face, but she could see that they were wearing a long white coat, and a strange, wide-brimmed hat.

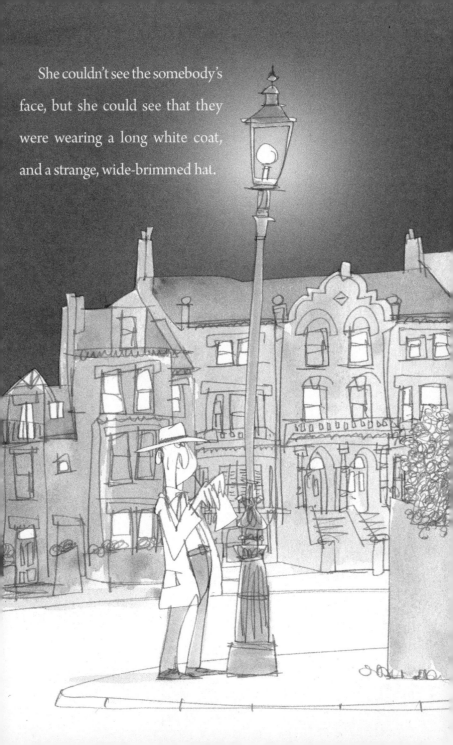

She watched as a large hand reached up to the poster, examined it for a moment and pulled it down. Then the somebody folded the poster into their pocket and, as if reacting to her presence, looked up at Imogen's bedroom window. For a split second, she could make out a man's face, and she ducked down beneath the curtains.

When Imogen looked back a few moments later, the man was gone.

CHAPTER SEVEN

Arthur's Revenge

The school playing fields were always muddy when it rained, and it had rained all week: that particularly cross sort of rain that melts the snow and then the grass beneath it too. The Year Two boys had spent the last hour doing football drills.

'Line up in your teams and practise passing!'

Mr Burnett, the coach, was standing at the edge of the football pitch in a full tracksuit, clutching a flask of hot coffee. 'Come on, Arthur!' he said. 'It isn't that cold!'

Arthur gave a particularly violent shiver and tried to dribble the ball towards his partner.

'You can go faster than that!' Mr Burnett cried.

Jack Jones sniggered and shoved Arthur out of the way. 'Move,' he said, and then dribbled the ball away across the grass, stopping here and there to bounce it in the air from foot to foot.

Arthur folded his arms. His trainers were muddy, and so were his knees. He was so muddy he felt like he might turn into mud, and have to squelch about on the football pitch for the rest of his life. At least mud didn't have to play football, though, so maybe it would be all right – as long as he didn't get stuck to Jack Jones's knees or anything like that.

'Are you okay?'

It was Theo.

'I'm fine,' said Arthur.

'Where's Einstein?' asked Theo.

'He's hiding inside. The mud messes up his feathers.

And I think he's still sad about his friend.'

Jack kicked the ball back to Arthur hard, so that it bashed him in the shins.

'Sir, sir! Arthur's not concentrating!' Jack whined.

'Arthur Stewart!' said Mr Burnett, marching over to stare down at him through a cloud of coffee steam. 'You might just be the worst footballer I've ever seen.'

Arthur looked down at his shoes and tried to laugh. 'Sorry, sir,' he mumbled.

'Don't worry,' whispered Theo. 'He said that to my brother last week.'.

Then Mr Burnett blew his orange whistle and started shouting. 'Right! Inside! Change and shower! Arthur, collect the cones! Jack, you're on balls! Theo, you help them out!'

A few minutes later, Arthur, Theo and Jack Jones were heading inside together through the drizzle. Most of the other boys had finished changing and were starting to disappear from the cloakroom, which was damp and smelly now, with clumps of mud all over the floor.

'Hi, Einstein,' said Theo very quietly.

Einstein was hiding inside Arthur's kitbag, doing his best not to squawk at the dirty football socks that had suddenly appeared beside him.

Arthur grinned, and opened the bag just wide enough for Theo to give Einstein a quick pat on the head.

'What are you two looking at?' said Jack.

Arthur zipped the bag up and turned round. 'Nothing.'

'*Nothing*,' Jack imitated. 'What's in your bag?'

Theo and Arthur glanced at each other.

'It's just a photo,' said Theo. 'Nothing interesting.'

'Let me see,' said Jack.

Arthur tried not to make eye contact. 'No,' he said.

'Why not?' Jack asked. 'If it's just a photo, why can't I see it?'

'Just show him the picture,' Theo whispered.

Arthur frowned. He didn't suppose it would do any harm, and it might stop Jack grabbing the bag off him and finding Einstein. He reached into the pocket of his backpack and pulled out the second Polaroid of Isaac.

Jack grabbed it. He frowned, and then sniggered. 'You keep a photo of a penguin at a zoo in your pocket? You're so weird.' He shoved the photo back into Arthur's hands and retreated to his corner of the changing room.

Arthur stared dumbly at the floor. 'A zoo . . .' he whispered to himself. Of course, the photo of Isaac had *obviously* been taken at a zoo. The water in the background didn't look natural at all. He'd been so distracted by what Isaac looked like in the photo that he'd forgotten to think about where it had actually been taken. He'd have to tell Imogen.

Arthur washed the dirt off his legs and got dressed

quickly. It was almost the end of the school day. In just a few minutes he'd be able to go home, and not have to worry about anything – not maths, not Jack Jones, not football, not Mr Burnett – for three entire weeks, until January. And, come January, Arthur felt convinced that he'd be far too grown up to ever need to worry about anything again.

He put his bag over his shoulder, waited for Theo to finish changing and turned to leave.

'Nice glasses,' someone sniggered.

It was Jack again. Arthur ignored him.

'Where are you two going?' asked Jack.

'Home,' said Arthur. He felt Einstein give an angry wriggle inside his bag.

'Are you going to tell your mummy I was mean to you?' Jack teased.

'Go away, Jack,' said Arthur quietly.

He hated it when this happened. He didn't like Jack, either, so what did it matter if Jack didn't like him? But

Jack always had quick things to say, and Arthur never did. His brain would stop working and his neck would go hot, and then he'd look stupid and babyish, just like Jack said he was.

'Crybaby,' Jack sniggered, and he pushed past to leave first.

'Unzip the bag,' whispered Theo.

'What?' said Arthur.

Einstein was still wriggling desperately from somewhere underneath Arthur's dirty football kit.

'Unzip it,' said Theo again.

Arthur shrugged and did as Theo said. No sooner had he opened it than Einstein burst from the bag and leaped spectacularly through the air – right towards Jack's head.

'Aaah!' Jack screamed, covering his face with his hands. 'Get off! Get off!'

Einstein had landed on Jack's shoulder and was angrily pecking his ears.

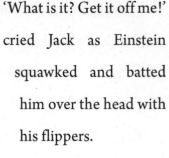

'What is it? Get it off me!' cried Jack as Einstein squawked and batted him over the head with his flippers.

The door of the changing room burst open. Hearing the footsteps, Einstein hopped down to the ground. Theo scooped him up and quickly hid him back inside Arthur's kitbag.

Mr Burnett came striding round the corner, his mouth already going flat at the corners like it did when he was about to tell someone off. 'What's going on in here, then?'

'It was Arthur!' Jack whimpered.

Arthur blinked nervously.

'Arthur?' said Mr Burnett sternly. 'What did you do?'

'Nothing,' said Arthur, not strictly telling a lie. 'I was just standing here.'

'There was a penguin!' said Jack desperately. 'He attacked me with a penguin!'

'A penguin?' Mr Burnett looked blankly from Arthur to Theo, as if waiting for one of them to fill him in.

'I don't know what he's talking about,' said Arthur. 'He just started yelling.'

Theo shrugged. 'I didn't see a penguin, either, sir. Do you think maybe he needs to go to the nurse?'

Mr Burnett frowned and shook his head. 'Get out, all of you.'

'I'm not making it up!' said Jack. 'He made a penguin appear!'

'That is *enough*!' said Mr Burnett, pleased at finally having something to raise his voice to. 'No more talking nonsense, or you'll be waiting on the edge of the pitch during football next term.'

'Sorry,' Jack mumbled, quickly falling silent. He picked his bag up from where he had dropped it and hurried out of the room.

'Maybe I'll start talking nonsense too if that's the punishment,' said Arthur to Theo, as they followed Jack outside.

It was still drizzling out in the playground, and the grey clouds had drooped a little closer to the ground. Arthur put his hood up as they walked towards the crowd of parents who were waiting, under a swarm of umbrellas, at the gates.

Just then Imogen came bursting out of the door of the library and hurried over to join them. Her hair was looking messier than usual, and she was clutching her ragged notebook to her chest.

'Hello,' she said, falling into step beside her brother.

'Hi?' said Arthur. Imogen was using her mysterious voice again.

'I've made several new discoveries,' she whispered.

'I'll explain everything when I can.'

'So have I!' said Arthur, pleased to finally be of use. 'Why can't you explain everything now?'

'Because we don't know who's listening!' Imogen gave the empty pavement a significant glance, shoved her notebook into her coat pocket and darted off again, as if she didn't really know them.

'Is your sister okay?' asked Theo.

Arthur shrugged. 'I don't know. She was acting crazy at breakfast too. It's about this friend of Einstein's.'

Einstein gave a sudden, sad little caw from inside Arthur's bag.

'Well?' said Imogen, shortly after supper that evening.

Just like they always did on the first night of the holidays, Imogen and Arthur had chosen a Christmas film to watch with their favourite pudding, which was apple crumble and ice cream. Mr Stewart had paused *The Grinch* and headed into the kitchen in order to pour what must have been his eleventh cup of tea.

'Well, what?' said Arthur.

'Well, what was your discovery?'

'I think Einstein and Isaac must have come from a zoo,' Arthur whispered, as their father sat back down in his armchair and pressed PLAY again on the remote control.

Imogen frowned. 'But Einstein's from Australia.'

'Aren't there zoos in Australia?'

Imogen hadn't thought about that. She'd been imagining vast plains and dramatic beaches.

'The background in the photo doesn't look natural,' Arthur went on.

'You might be right,' Imogen admitted. She actually sounded impressed.

'And what was your discovery?' Arthur asked.

Imogen thought about the man she had seen on the street outside. It hardly seemed real now, in front of the telly with her family all around her. Maybe she'd been dreaming, after all – and anyway she didn't want

Arthur worrying about it and telling their parents.

'Nothing yet,' she said quietly. 'I'm still thinking.'

'Oh,' said Arthur. 'Well, shall we tell Mum and Dad that we think Einstein's from a zoo?'

'No,' said Imogen sharply. 'Dad will want to send him back to it.'

'Shh,' said Mr Stewart, and Einstein – who was sitting on his lap – gave them a stroppy little squawk too. 'We're trying to watch *The Grinch*.'

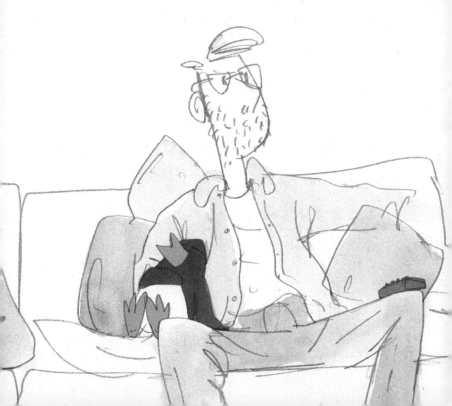

Imogen and Arthur looked at each other and tried not to giggle.

They stayed like that for the rest of the film. Mr Stewart didn't even look cross when Einstein fell asleep and started to snore like a foghorn, and Imogen watched them and thought about how maybe – just maybe – if Mr Stewart was getting used to Einstein, he would get used to a second penguin too, and everything would be okay.

Their parents let them stay awake for a whole hour beyond their usual bedtime. Then, spotting the time on the clock above the fireplace, Mrs Stewart clapped her hands together and cried, 'Quick – straight to bed! Or you'll be much too tired for our shopping trip tomorrow.'

As they walked up the stairs, Arthur managed to give Imogen a brief, whispered, blow-by-blow account of Einstein's daring battle with Jack Jones.

'If Mr Burnett hadn't come in, he would probably

have killed him,' Arthur exaggerated, and, in the dazed sleepiness brought on by apple crumble, he almost believed it.

*

Christmas holidays or not, Imogen couldn't sleep.

She could hear Arthur snoring next door, and her parents listening to the news downstairs with the volume low. The streetlamps outside were casting narrow shadows through the blinds the way they always did after lights-out. Imogen stared up at the ceiling, with all its luminous star stickers and bits of old Blu-tack, and thought about Isaac again.

What would a *real* detective do? She had put up posters, she had written everything she knew down in a notebook, she had looked at things through a magnifying glass – but what now? Isaac's crate hadn't even had a proper address on it: he could be anywhere in the UK. He could have been shipped off to another country altogether. What were the chances of someone identifying him from some posters on a few little streets in London? The strange man in the hat had seemed interested in their posters, of course – perhaps he knew something. Or perhaps he was an assassin, or a penguin-murderer, or whatever kind of person it is that stuffs animals before they go on display in museums.

'Check the newspapers!' she breathed suddenly, sitting up in bed.

How could she have been so stupid? It was what Inspector Bucket did when things went missing: he would check all the papers for any events that might give him some sort of clue – like when a painting went missing from a gallery in London, and he had found the thief trying to sell it through a newspaper advertisement in Bristol. Of course, it would be easier for Imogen because Inspector Bucket lived in the olden days and didn't have the internet.

She grabbed her notebook, jumped into her

fluffy slippers, and tiptoed down the corridor to the computer in Mrs Stewart's study.

Imogen sat down at her mother's desk, opened the laptop and bit her lip in thought. She tried typing **lost pengwin** into Google, but nothing useful came up – just a few silly-looking storybooks. Then she tried **missing pengwin**, **kidnapped pengwin** and **pengwin escape**. Several articles appeared:

Penguin Escape Plan Foiled By Zoo Workers...

Penguin Stolen From Dublin Zoo Safely Returned...
Lost Penguin's Daring Escape From Sydney Zoo Filmed On...

Imogen breathed in sharply. Sydney: that had been on Einstein's flight label. She opened the article and scrolled down the page:

Lost Penguin's Daring Escape From Sydney Zoo Filmed On CCTV (27th November)

A little penguin from Sydney Zoo – known by his keepers as Einstein – managed to escape from Sydney Zoo on Wednesday. Zookeeper Ted Smith reported that Einstein had been visibly restless since the transportation of one of Sydney Zoo's rockhopper penguins to a zoo in the UK a few weeks beforehand. It is unclear whether this detail influenced Einstein's escape, but when a gate in the enclosure was left open during feeding time Einstein made a dash for freedom, and was quickly lost among the crowds. His initial escape from the penguin enclosure was caught on CCTV, but the zoo has so far been unable to find out how, and indeed if, he managed to escape from the zoo itself.

If anyone has any information relating to the location of Einstein the penguin, they should contact Sydney Zoo immediately. Einstein is particularly distinctive due to his orange beak, which differs from the standard dark beak of other little penguins. This mutation helps his zookeepers to recognise him.

Little penguins, otherwise known as fairy penguins, are the world's smallest penguin species, growing up to around 34 cm and weighing up to 1.4 kg . . .

*

So Arthur had been right.

Imogen's heart was pounding. She opened a new tab and quickly searched for **rockhopper pengwins UK.**

The first result was Edinburgh Zoo, the second London – but Einstein had been to London Zoo already. The penguins in the pictures had red eyes and spiky yellow eyebrows, just like Isaac's. One of them – the smallest – looked exactly like her photo, right down to the last feather. Could it be Isaac?

Imogen grabbed her notebook and scribbled down her findings, underlining Edinburgh, Sydney and Einstein in her mother's red biro.

'Rachel – you've left the light on in your study!' Mr Stewart's voice sounded from the staircase.

Imogen's eyes widened and she slammed the laptop shut.

'Oh, have I?' Mrs Stewart replied. 'Can you get it for me?'

'All right.' Her father's footsteps started to approach along the corridor.

Imogen jumped up from the desk and rushed over to the door, then stood with her back pressed against it, holding her breath as she thought of excuses.

I forgot I needed to use the internet for my homework – would that work? On the first night of the school holidays?

The creaky floorboard outside the door went *creak!* – and Imogen prepared herself for a telling-off – when suddenly—

'James! Can you help me find the front-door keys?' Mrs Stewart called up the stairs. 'I need to lock up.'

Mr Stewart paused. Imogen could hear him moving on the other side of the door, which was still slightly ajar.

His hand reached blindly through the gap and flicked the light switch beside her head, and then he turned round. She breathed out as she heard his footsteps retreating along the corridor and down the stairs.

'I think they're next to the kettle!' he said.

Seizing the moment, Imogen opened the door of the study and scampered along the corridor as quickly and quietly as she could, taking extra care as she passed the stairwell. She opened the door of her bedroom, tucked her notebook underneath an old teddy bear and dived into bed. And, after her mind had stopped racing, she fell asleep, feeling very much like a detective.

CHAPTER EIGHT

Christmas Shopping

Central London was fizzing with Christmas lights. There was something about school having broken up that made the streets feel bright and sparkling no matter how dull the sky was, like Christmas didn't need to prove itself any more. Imogen kept Einstein in her pocket and had to be dragged away from almost every shop window they walked past – with all the tinsel and fake snow, even supermarkets and unfashionable clothing stores for old men seemed suddenly fascinating.

Arthur was less keen on busy streets. He liked the decorations too, but for Arthur being in a crowd was a little like being underwater. He kept hold of Mrs Stewart's hand and tried to avoid the tourists who weaved about him in directionless lines and paused in difficult places to put up umbrellas. Each time a taxi or bus came whooshing past, the buildings looming overhead would seem suddenly taller and more menacing.

'Here we are,' said Mrs Stewart, steering him left into a great big department store.

They stood still at last to ride the escalator, and Arthur breathed a sigh of relief. As he watched all the baubles floating past in pretty colours, it was finally quiet enough to remember what Imogen was so excited about.

'Imogen!' he said. 'Make sure Einstein gets to see the decorations!'

But Einstein was one step ahead of him, and was

already trying to remove a string of tinsel from the edge of the escalator with his beak.

'Einstein, no!' said Imogen. She leaped to the other side of the escalator so that Einstein could no longer reach it, but rather than forcing him to let go, as she'd hoped, the sudden movement only caused Einstein to tug harder. All at once, the whole string of tinsel from the left-hand side of the escalator broke free from where it was fastened. Imogen, Arthur and Mrs Stewart watched as it tumbled, sparkling red, to land with an echoing flop on the ground floor below.

They looked at each other for a moment, wide-eyed. Then, 'Quick, run!' Mrs Stewart cried, and she started to rush up the remainder of the escalator.

'Where to?' said Arthur, bounding up the steps to keep up with her.

'I don't know! Into a shop!' she said. 'And give me that penguin, Imogen!'

Einstein honked indignantly as Mrs Stewart grabbed him out of Imogen's pocket and shoved him sideways into her handbag.

'We are just a normal family,' Mrs Stewart hissed, taking each of her children by the hand and leading them into the first shop they came across. 'Walking very casually into a men's clothing store.'

Einstein gave a wriggle from inside her handbag, squawked sulkily, poked the fabric once with his flipper and reluctantly settled down.

'Ooh, do you think Dad would like this for Christmas, Imogen?' said Mrs Stewart, raising her voice back to a normal volume as she examined a leather satchel.

'He already has one a bit like that,' said Imogen.

'That's how we know he'd like it . . .' said Mrs Stewart. 'But what about this scarf?'

'I thought we were going to the toyshop,' said Arthur sulkily.

'Not until we've picked out presents for Dad and your grandparents.'

'Maybe they'd like toys too?'

'You'll get toys for Christmas, Arthur,' said Imogen, feeling particularly grown up all of a sudden. 'Stop being such a baby.'

Eventually they settled on a nice new belt for Mr Stewart, and some woolly gloves to send to their grandfather. Imogen hadn't yet found a moment to tell her brother about last night's discovery, and tried to get his attention several times as they walked through the department store towards the toyshop. But Arthur was in a sulk with her, and pretended to be far too interested in his own shoes to notice when she said his name.

'Arthur,' said Imogen, for the third time. 'I have to tell you something.'

'Why would you have to tell me something if I'm only a baby?' said Arthur.

'Well, you *definitely* sound like one now!' said Imogen.

'Stop bickering,' said Mrs Stewart. 'Let's just pop into the food section to get some of those ginger biscuits Granny likes.'

'The food section smells like fish,' Arthur grumbled.

The entrance did smell like fish, but beyond the fish counters were various stalls piled high with cakes and chocolates. Suddenly Imogen and Arthur were far too busy working out how many they could buy with their pocket money to remember they had fallen out. The chocolates were all very expensive, though, and after last week's cupcake purchase Imogen only had 20p left in her pocket. Luckily the man behind the counter let them both have a free sample, and didn't even mind when Imogen said vaguely, 'They're lovely! We might buy some later . . .' and then quickly shuffled off.

'Anyway,' said Imogen, as Arthur stood on his

tiptoes and glanced around to see where Mrs Stewart had got to, 'I think Isaac's in Edinburgh.'

Arthur looked at her. 'Why?'

'I found a news article. They're from Sydney Zoo, both of them. And then Isaac was moved to a zoo somewhere in the UK. The article didn't say which zoo, but Einstein already checked if Isaac was in London. And there's a picture of a rockhopper penguin in Edinburgh that looks exactly like Isaac.'

'What's a rockhopper penguin?'

'The sort of penguin Isaac is.'

'So what do we do?' asked Arthur.

'I don't know,' said Imogen. She bit her lip seriously. 'Maybe we'll have to run away.'

'Why don't we just tell Mum and Dad?'

It had never really occurred to Imogen that she could *tell* her parents something like that, and she considered it for a moment – but of course it still wouldn't work. Mr Stewart had always made it clear that Einstein was only staying until they found out where his real home was.

'If we tell them that Einstein comes from Sydney Zoo, then they'll call the zoo and send him home!' Imogen pointed out, her stomach sinking as she said it. 'People from the zoo are probably already looking for him. Mum will think it's wrong to keep him a secret and then—'

'Imogen! Arthur!'

Suddenly Mrs Stewart appeared beside them with the box of ginger biscuits in her hand. She looked frantic. 'I've lost him!'

'*What?*'

'I noticed when I was getting my purse out! He's gone from my handbag! Einstein!'

'How can he be gone?' said Arthur.

'Do you think they arrested him for breaking the tinsel?' said Imogen.

Then, all at once, everyone remembered.

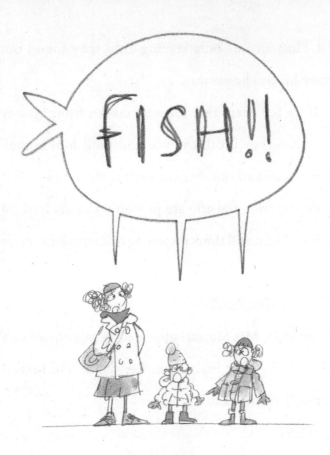

'Fish!' they cried in unison, and turned to run towards the entrance of the food hall.

Mrs Stewart headed for the door, where the view was best, while Imogen ran towards the fish counters and Arthur, being the smallest, crouched down to look around for penguins hiding at knee height.

'I can't see him!' cried Imogen, pushing past a disgruntled pair of old men who had been asking about some expensive-looking salmon. She glanced desperately up and down the ice-filled glass cases. It was Einstein's idea of heaven: he could be anywhere. But she was met only with the slimy, silvery stare of row upon row of cold, dead fish. Imogen shuddered and turned away.

She looked up at the person standing closest to her. 'Excuse me, have you seen a—'

Imogen froze. It was him: it was the man who had taken her poster down – she was sure of it. He was real, after all, and he was still dressed in his hat and long white coat, and he was peering down at her with great interest.

'A what, love?' he prompted.

Perhaps he *did* know something, but looking up at his face Imogen felt quite certain – with the sort of gut feeling Inspector Bucket liked to work on – that this was not a man she could trust. There was something about the way his eyebrow arched as he looked at her, about the serious lines in his oddly pale face.

'A cat,' she finished faintly.

The man looked surprised. 'No, I haven't seen any cats,' he said.

'Don't worry,' said Imogen, smiling quickly. 'Thank you for your help!' She pushed past him and ran back towards her brother.

'Have you seen him?' said Arthur, standing up from the floor.

'No, have you?' Imogen's heart was pounding. She was still looking out for Einstein, but she couldn't stop glancing over at the man. And she had the horrible feeling that he was watching her back.

'I can't,' said Arthur. 'There's too many people.' It was true: the black and white tiled floor that seemed to stretch endlessly around them was covered in people, and entirely empty of penguins.

'There!' cried Imogen. Across the hall, a woman in

an apron and a funny straw hat was wheeling several crates of fish along behind the counters. Just for a moment, Imogen thought she saw a dark blue flipper poke through one of the gaps.

'Where?' said Arthur.

She glanced over at where the man in the white coat had been standing – good, he had turned round. 'Follow me!'

Imogen led the way as they pushed through the crowd back to the fish counters. 'Excuse me!' she said, as they reached the lady in the straw hat.

The woman paused and looked down at the two small children, who were both panting and looking flustered. 'Yes?'

'I'd like to see your fish, please,' said Imogen, through another pant.

'There's fish on the counters,' said the woman, and started to walk away again.

'No, no, wait!' cried Imogen. 'I'd like to see *your* fish.'

'*My* fish?'

'What I mean is,' said Imogen, 'are you sure that's *fish* in there?'

'Look – do you kids have an adult with you or should I call security?'

'There!' shouted Arthur, tugging on Imogen's sleeve and pointing desperately at the bottom crate. 'I saw his arm!'

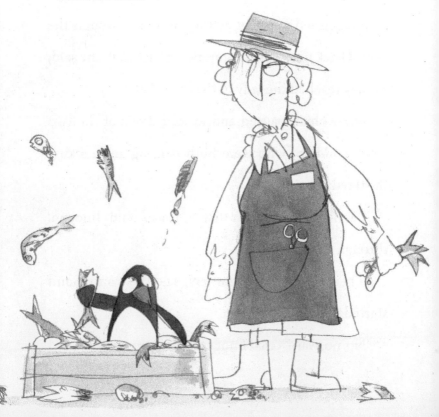

'An arm?!' The woman in the funny hat looked horrified, and started to quickly unload the crates from her trolley.

'I mean flipper,' said Arthur.

The woman lifted the second-to-last crate, and up popped Einstein's head.

'Einstein!' cried Imogen.

Einstein squawked sheepishly and let her pick him up. Imogen wiped the fish scales off his feathers with her coat sleeve, patted him on the head and put him back in her pocket.

'Phew,' she said. 'Can you see Mum, Arthur?'

Then they remembered the woman.

She was staring down at them, her eyebrows raised so high that it looked like her straw hat was about to pop off the top of her head. Imogen stared back, and then all three of them turned to the crate they had pulled Einstein out of.

It was a mess. Half the fish were gone, and the rest were pecked to pieces.

'He's gone and eaten all my sardines!' said the woman.

Imogen and Arthur looked at each other.

'We have to go,' said Arthur.

'I should probably call security . . .' said the woman, frowning.

'And we should probably go,' said Imogen, backing away as the woman's disbelief started to turn, very slowly, to anger.

'Will Mum have to pay?' asked Arthur, as they quickly walked towards the door.

'I don't know,' said Imogen, and they broke into a run.

'Mum!'

'Arthur!' Mrs Stewart was still looking around near the entrance. 'Have you found him?'

'He's in my coat,' said Imogen. 'We need to go!'

'Why? What's happened?' asked Mrs Stewart, but she knew not to stick around to find out.

They all hurried over to the escalator. Then, just as Imogen was about to jump on to it, she crashed into someone, who stumbled and dropped the pieces of paper he'd been holding.

'Sorry,' said Imogen, and quickly bent down to pick up his things. 'Hang on,' she frowned. At the top of the pile was a picture of Einstein and Isaac, and underneath that a cutout of the very newspaper article she had discovered last night.

Her cheeks burned red as she looked up, but she already knew whose face she was going to see: it was the same man again. Mrs Stewart and Arthur had disappeared down the escalator. They wouldn't be able to see her, and they wouldn't be able to see him, either.

'Sorry, dear,' the man began, reaching out a hand to take the photos back from her. 'That was my fault

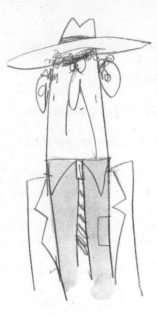

really. I wasn't looking.' He spoke in a mild Australian accent: she hadn't noticed that before.

Imogen took a step backwards, gaping at him like a fish.

'Can I have those back? They're very important.' He came closer, still holding out his hand.

'No!' shouted Imogen, so loudly that even she was surprised by the sound of her own voice, and she darted away from him and hurried down the escalator, following the red streak of colour that was Mrs Stewart's coat – just as it disappeared on to the street outside.

They were hailing a taxi when Imogen caught up with them.

'What about the toyshop?' said Arthur hopefully, as they clambered in. But he didn't really mean it.

Imogen sank down into her seat, avoiding the

window, and she kept her breath held until the taxi had pulled away from the pavement and joined the nameless flood of traffic heading out of central London.

CHAPTER NINE

A Difficult Decision

Imogen turned the man's newspaper cutout over in her hands and looked at it again.

Lost Penguin's Daring Escape From Sydney Zoo Filmed On CCTV

Some bullet points were scrawled in black pen in the margin, listing Einstein's flight details. Further down the page, the man seemed to have come to the same conclusion that she had:

LOOKING FOR ISAAC - EDINBURGH?

She folded it back over and shuddered. It all seemed so sinister all of a sudden. What did the man want with Einstein? What did he want with Isaac? And, if *he* knew Isaac was in Edinburgh, what was to stop him from getting there first? All the sorts of criminals Imogen had read about in her detective books came flooding through her head. Perhaps he was an art thief: she didn't think art thieves had much interest in penguins, but you never could tell with villains. Or maybe a kidnapper? That seemed likely: kidnappers would probably kidnap anyone they could get their hands on, penguin or otherwise.

Even so, she didn't know how to find and rescue Isaac without asking her parents for help and, if she did ask them for help, she'd have to tell them the truth about where Einstein had come from. And then they'd send him home to Sydney. But if she did nothing? Imogen didn't know what would happen if she did nothing, but she had a terrible feeling about it. The sort of feeling that makes your insides go all fidgety.

There was a small knock at her bedroom door.

'Come in!' Imogen said.

It was Arthur. Einstein waddled in after him.

'Mum wants to know if you want anything to eat,' said Arthur.

'I'm not hungry.'

Arthur frowned. 'Are you sure?' he asked. 'You're usually hungry.'

Imogen sat down on her bed. 'Well, I'm not hungry today. I have to think.'

'Are you thinking about your detective work?' asked Arthur.

'I don't know,' said Imogen. 'I'm not sure I want to be a detective any more.'

'But we're so close to finding Isaac!'

Einstein looked up and squawked in interest: now Arthur had given her away.

'I don't know, Einstein,' said Imogen apologetically. 'I think Isaac might be in Edinburgh, but I can't be sure without going there.'

'Have you got the picture of the penguin in Edinburgh?' said Arthur. 'Einstein will be able to tell if it's Isaac or not. Won't you, Einstein?'

Imogen's stomach did another somersault. She wasn't sure Arthur understood their problem, but she wasn't sure she had any other choice, either.

'Okay,' said Imogen. 'Get Mum's laptop and I'll show you the photo.'

Arthur hurried along the corridor and came back with the laptop a moment later. When Imogen opened it up and searched for the photo, Einstein erupted in such an excited flurry of squawks and clucks that Arthur had to slam the door shut to stop their parents from hearing.

'Shh,' said Imogen. 'Don't hit the screen with your flipper!'

Arthur grabbed the laptop off his sister and stared at it. 'Where's Einstein's photo of Isaac?' he asked, and Imogen took her detective notebook out of her dressing-gown pocket, opened it to the right page and handed it to him.

They set the two side by side, and looked from one to the other. It was just as Imogen had thought the night before: hard to tell, of course, but the feathers were the same – and, with Einstein's reaction, it was almost certain...

Then, leaning over with her pen, Imogen added to last week's spider diagram:

Isaac is definitely in Edinburgh.

Arthur grinned excitedly. 'So let's tell Mum and Dad. We need to go to Edinburgh and find him!'

Imogen nodded, but she seemed uncertain.

'What's wrong?' asked Arthur.

'If Mum and Dad find out where Einstein's really from, then they'll tell Sydney Zoo. What if he doesn't like living in a zoo?'

Arthur stopped grinning. 'We could leave that bit of the story out?' he suggested hopefully.

'But how can we tell them about Isaac without telling them everything else too? We'll have to show them the newspaper article just to persuade them we're not making it up.'

'Well, maybe we can convince Mum and Dad to let us keep him anyway,' said Arthur.

'Maybe,' Imogen agreed, but she didn't really think so. Even if Mr and Mrs Stewart *wanted* to keep Einstein, there was no way they'd keep the story secret. It wasn't the sort of secret a grown-up would like to keep. Mr Stewart was too honest, and Mrs Stewart would worry too much. And, if Sydney Zoo wanted Einstein back, what was to stop them from taking the penguin that was rightfully theirs?

'And if we *don't* ask them for help . . .' said Arthur.

'Then I only have twenty pee and two paperclips in my moneybox, so we won't go to Edinburgh *or* find Isaac,' Imogen finished. 'And there's something else I haven't told you,' she said. 'I saw someone at the department store,' and she explained all about the strange man, and how he'd taken their poster down, and how he seemed to have followed them. She showed her brother the notes and the photos he had been carrying.

'So what does he want?' asked Arthur.

Imogen shook her head. 'I don't know,' she said. 'But he's clearly looking for Isaac too.'

'Then we have to go!' said Arthur. 'What if he wants to hurt Isaac? We have to stop him!'

Einstein honked.

Imogen nodded. 'I know,' she said. 'But what if

he's in Edinburgh when we get there? And what if he wants to hurt Einstein too?'

'Then we'll fight him!' said Arthur. He thought about Einstein pecking Jack Jones's ears in the changing room at school, and felt suddenly much braver than usual.

Imogen knew that he was right. There wasn't any other choice – and, besides, it seemed fitting that she, a detective, should have an arch-nemesis on her trail. It made her feel important, as well as a little scared.

'You're right. We don't have to tell Mum and Dad that bit about the strange man, though.'

'Why not?'

'Because they might not let us go to Edinburgh if they really think it's dangerous.' She left a dramatic pause, just for effect. 'This is something we need to sort out for ourselves.'

'What do you think, Einstein?' Arthur asked. 'We're a family now, aren't we?'

Einstein looked up sadly from the laptop screen and nodded.

'But he only met us because he was looking for Isaac. That's why he's really here,' said Imogen. 'Squawk once if you want to go to Edinburgh and find Isaac, and twice if you don't.'

There was a long silence. Einstein stared at the laptop screen, and then up at his human friends. Then he gave a long, single squawk.

CHAPTER TEN

Train to Edinburgh

After they had told their parents everything, Imogen felt ashamed that she had ever been indecisive. After all, she'd always known that Einstein's time with them was temporary. She had just convinced herself that they might be able to keep him forever. But he wasn't like one of her toys, was he? He was a real penguin, with real penguin friends and a real penguin family, even if they were from a zoo. All she had done was make everything harder for herself – and for Arthur too.

Still, she couldn't help but feel nervous about it. The strange man's notes had *said* Edinburgh on them. She kept imagining walking up to the zoo and finding him waiting there with a net, ready to steal Einstein away from her.

'Cheer up, Im!' said Mr Stewart, as he shoved their overnight bags into the back of the taxi. 'We're going on an adventure!'

Of course, her father couldn't possibly understand the seriousness of the situation. As far as Imogen could tell, Mr Stewart was viewing their trip to Edinburgh as some sort of holiday. She sighed crossly and brushed her hair out of her face. She would have to be the responsible one yet again: grown-ups never understood anything.

'I don't know what you're so happy about, James,' said Mrs Stewart. All day at home she had hardly been able to sit down for five minutes without springing up to check the answer machine or peer anxiously out of the window.

'Neither do I,' said Mr Stewart amusedly. 'Although I suppose now that we're going to Edinburgh, we might stop the police from finding us and pressing charges for damaged tinsel?'

'James, that is *not* funny!'

Mr Stewart chuckled and sat down beside her in the back of the taxi. Arthur and Imogen took the two fold-down seats that faced the back. It was late evening, and they both looked tired. Arthur snuggled Einstein close to his chest and fell into a light doze as the taxi started to move.

The driver eyed Einstein suspiciously through the rear-view mirror. 'They make them very realistic these days, don't they?' he said.

Mrs Stewart laughed awkwardly and said something about the weather.

'Anyway,' she went on, 'if the children are right about Einstein being from Sydney Zoo, imagine what will happen if someone who recognises him sees yesterday's CCTV footage from the department store?'

Imogen thought about the man again. Had he seen the footage? Did he know Einstein was with them, or did he only suspect it?

'I don't know,' said Mr Stewart blankly. 'What *will* happen?'

'Well, I think the whole thing's a bit far-fetched,' Mrs Stewart sniffed. 'I don't know why we're humouring Imogen's conspiracy theories.'

'I am a professional detective!' Imogen protested, but she was only half listening, and quickly went back to watching two pigeons on the street outside fighting over a soggy-looking crisp.

Mr Stewart shrugged. 'The whole thing was pretty ridiculous in the first place, though, wasn't it? No harm in accepting a bit *more* ridiculousness now that we've started.'

'If we all accepted that as a principle, then the

whole world would have gone mad years ago!'

'You're the one who's been cooking gourmet meals for a penguin, dear.'

Mrs Stewart sniffed again and checked her watch. 'The last train to Edinburgh leaves in twenty minutes,' she said. 'Let's hope the traffic's good.'

They had meant to leave with more time to spare, but getting everyone out of the house was always challenging. As soon as one person had found their shoes, someone else would have lost theirs, and then the cat would want feeding and the bathroom door would get stuck, and then all of a sudden it was past ten o'clock and the sleeper train's departure time was approaching fast.

On top of that, Mr and Mrs Stewart kept bickering and changing their minds.

'He's officially a missing penguin,' Mr Stewart had said, after seeing Imogen's newspaper article. 'We can't just take him to Edinburgh! We need to report this straight away.'

'Oh, but how would you feel if *you* were all alone in a strange place, looking for a long-lost friend?' Mrs Stewart had retorted. 'Would *you* want to be packed off home?'

Then, every few minutes, they would swap. 'I just don't know if we should be doing this . . .' Mrs Stewart would mutter under her breath. And all of a sudden everyone was arguing again.

'Stop it!' Arthur had shouted eventually. It was usually Imogen who did the shouting, so the shock of it made them all fall silent. 'Einstein has come all the way across the world to find his friend! Are you really going to stop him at the last minute just because you can't stop arguing?'

Einstein followed this with a loud squawk, for good measure.

'No, you're right . . .' Mr Stewart muttered awkwardly. 'I'd better phone a taxi.'

The taxi got caught in several traffic lights near the station. Mr Stewart couldn't stop checking his watch and peering anxiously out of the window. Eventually he got fed up.

'Don't worry about parking, we'll get out here,' he told the driver, and handed the money over with a tip.

Of course, he was only worried about losing money on the train tickets, Imogen thought to herself. But she was glad to see him hurry all the same.

'Why aren't we parking?' asked Arthur sleepily.

'We're going to have to run for it.'

Mr and Mrs Stewart jumped out and grabbed the bags from the back, and Imogen and Arthur followed them out on to the dark, drizzling street. Imogen was starting to feel very sleepy too. When her father shouted, 'Let's go!' and everyone rushed towards the station, she felt a bit like she was running in her sleep.

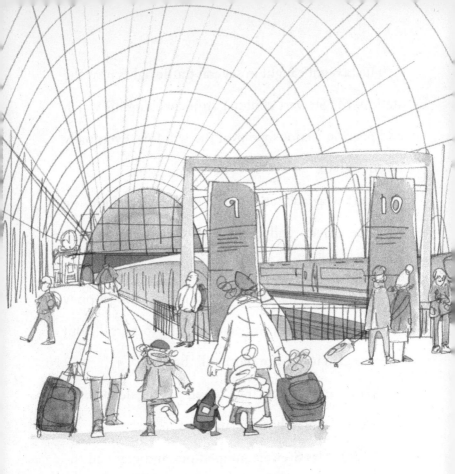

It was late, so the platform was mostly empty. Mrs Stewart quickly checked the departures board and they ran towards the waiting train, which was just about ready to leave. One of the conductors on the platform tutted as Mr Stewart slammed the button to open the carriage.

'Ten seconds later and you'd have missed it!' he said.

Imogen and Mrs Stewart jumped on to the train, and Mr Stewart turned round to wait for Arthur, who was just behind them. Keeping hold of Einstein had slowed him down a little.

'Come on,' said Mr Stewart, reaching out his hand.

Suddenly Arthur froze.

'Come *on!*' said Mr Stewart.

'That doesn't say Edinburgh!' said Arthur, staring up at the screen beside the train. The lenses of his glasses were spattered with raindrops, and he wasn't quite sure how to spell 'Edinburgh' anyway, but he was sure it wasn't spelled like *that*. 'You're on the wrong train!'

Mr Stewart's eyes widened as he saw what the screen said too. 'Imogen! Rachel! Get off the train! This one's going to Liverpool!'

They jumped back down to the platform just as the

train doors hissed to a close behind them.

'Which one is it?!' cried Imogen.

'Edinburgh's platform six, not nine,' said the same conductor who had tutted at them a moment earlier. He checked his watch. 'You won't make it.'

Mrs Stewart grabbed hold of Einstein, Mr Stewart picked up Arthur, and everyone ran as fast as they possibly could to platform six. Imogen was pretty sure no other nine-year-old had run so quickly before, and that, if only Mr Burnett had seen her, she'd have been made captain of every team in school.

They jumped on to the train with seconds to spare.

It took a while to find the right compartment. Mr Stewart had made everyone jump into the first carriage they could reach, but the one with their rooms in was all the way at the front of the train. They walked down the narrow corridors as the train started to rumble and move beneath them, slowly winding its way out of London.

It was a biggish compartment, with two bunk beds at either end. Imogen had secretly imagined something grander: she'd never been on a sleeper train before, and thought of them as being like trains from the olden days, with polished wood and chandeliers, whereas this one looked quite modern and ordinary. Arthur didn't mind, though. He was too busy claiming the top bunk for himself and Einstein.

'I get the top bunk, remember?' said Imogen.

Arthur looked blank. 'But I got here first,' he said.

Imogen raised an eyebrow at him, and suddenly he remembered.

'But that only applies to cars!' said Arthur, in protest.

'*Dad!*' Imogen started. 'Guess what Arthur did last—'

'Okay, fine!' said Arthur, and he hopped back down, looking sulky.

'Straight to sleep,' said Mrs Stewart. 'When you

wake up, we'll be in Edinburgh!'

Although she was tired, Imogen didn't drift off straight away. She lay still in the top bunk, watching light move through the chink in the blinds, and listening to her parents whispering on the other side of the compartment. Sometimes the light would shine through two chinks at once and she thought it looked like dragon eyes blinking at her.

Arthur gave Einstein his second pillow, and made sure to lend him a corner of duvet too. Soon they left London behind, and the light stopped flickering in quite so often. And so they fell asleep to the gentle rumbling of the train tracks, and the pattering of rain against the roof.

CHAPTER ELEVEN

Detective Bill Hunter

It was hardly morning when the train pulled into Edinburgh Waverley Station.

They had been woken up half an hour beforehand by a loud lady with a trolley of breakfast things. Arthur was far too excited to mind that it was early, and quickly sprang to life.

'Is that a dog?' said the trolley-lady, catching a glimpse of Einstein beneath the covers as Arthur threw back his duvet.

Arthur went pink. 'Oh – er ...'

'It's all right,' said the lady. 'They're allowed. Just keep him out of the bed, all right?'

Arthur nodded quickly.

Imogen felt it was far too early to be very hungry, and could only nibble on the corner of a dry-tasting shortbread. 'I don't like it,' she said eventually, and handed the rest to Arthur, who ate ten.

Mr Stewart sipped some black coffee while Mrs Stewart scrolled on her phone. 'Looks like the zoo won't be open yet,' she said. 'But we can go somewhere nice for breakfast first. If Arthur still has any room for breakfast, that is.'

It was a bright grey sort of day in Edinburgh. The sun started to rise shortly after they'd left the station, though you wouldn't have noticed if it wasn't for the fading darkness: the sky was one great cloud, without a gap in it to let a sunbeam through. Still, Arthur thought it suited the grey stone walls of the old buildings, and made the castle up on the hill look like something out of a storybook.

They found a café to sit down in for breakfast. Imogen had woken up enough to regain her appetite, and ate most of a stack of pancakes. Arthur, still full of shortbread, nibbled at the edges of the few she left, while Mr and Mrs Stewart had boring grown-up things like yoghurt and fruit.

'Do you have any raw herrings?' Mrs Stewart asked the waitress, when she came over to check that everything was all right.

The waitress looked confused. 'Is this for you?'

'Oh, no,' Mrs Stewart laughed bashfully. 'Just for the penguin, of course!'

The waitress spotted Einstein sitting between the two children on the far side of the table and jumped. 'Oh!' she said, and shook her head slightly, as if to check she was really awake. 'No . . . we don't have much call for raw herrings. But I could do kippers?'

'Ooh, could you do them with marmalade?' said Mrs Stewart. '*What*, James? He *likes* marmalade!'

'Sure,' said the waitress, and she wandered back to the kitchen in a daze.

Einstein gobbled up the first half of his plate of kippers in high spirits, but slowed down over the rest. Eventually he stopped eating altogether.

'Oh, dear,' said Mr Stewart dryly. 'Maybe he doesn't like the marmalade, after all.'

'He's just nervous,' Imogen explained.

She knew how he felt. Now that she'd finished her pancakes, she was feeling a little queasy too. What if Isaac wasn't there, after all, or that man had got to him first? And, even if Isaac was there, what would they do with him? They couldn't just steal him away from the zoo, could they? And she didn't suppose there was much chance of Edinburgh Zoo agreeing to send Isaac back to Sydney. They'd come such a long way just to see a penguin through the walls of an enclosure. Maybe their adventure would turn out to be a disappointing one.

'Are you okay?' Arthur asked his sister a little later as they wandered past the flamingoes on the way into the zoo.

'Of course,' said Imogen, and she gave him her reassuring smile.

Arthur was feeling pretty happy himself, but it made him nervous when Imogen went quiet. He was only her assistant, after all: she was the one who tended to notice things first. So, when she wore her thoughtful face, he worried that he had missed something obvious, like when he hadn't been able to see that Einstein's stay might be cut short by all this detective work. But he was trying not to think about that.

The zoo had only just opened, so it was still quiet, and they had a good view of all the animals they walked past. Mr Stewart made everyone stop at the flamingoes, and again at the red pandas, and again at the monkeys, until eventually Mrs Stewart got tired.

'Can we get on with seeing the penguins?' she said, rolling her eyes.

'The children like the monkeys,' said Mr Stewart defensively. 'No need to get impatient.' But he hurried up all the same.

As they turned the corner towards the penguin enclosure, Imogen's nervousness quickly turned to excitement. Einstein was tucked safely inside her coat. Arthur had wanted to keep Einstein inside

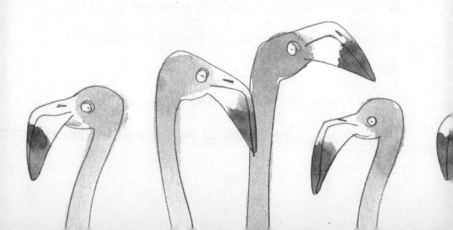

his own coat, but it was much smaller, so Einstein's flippers were in danger of poking out and giving them away.

'Remember, look for the ones with the spiky yellow eyebrows,' said Imogen, as she and Arthur started to run ahead of their parents.

'There's so many of them!' said Arthur.

The penguin enclosure was large. A great big lake stretched across it, with artificial beaches round the edges that sloped down into the water. Imogen and Arthur started by running over the bridge that went across the middle. There were penguins swimming

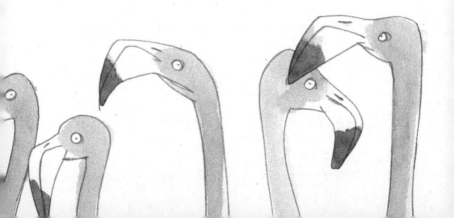

in the water underneath them, and more waddling about on the tarmac banks, but none of them looked like Isaac.

Arthur frowned and pulled himself up on the railings to get a better view. 'There!' he said.

'What?' said Imogen. 'I don't see anything!'

'On the far side of the lake! I thought I saw some with yellow eyebrows!'

He led the way. They ran across the bridge and followed a ramp down the side of the lake until they reached a small platform with glass walls that formed a window into the middle of the water. When Arthur stood on it, penguins swam past him at head height. The water was murky blue, and the birds appeared like shadows against it. He peered through the glass and tried to spot the penguin he had seen a moment ago.

'That was the one I saw,' said Arthur uncertainly.

'That's not Isaac,' said Imogen, but Arthur already

knew. This penguin's eyebrows were more white than yellow, and anyway it was too big.

Arthur sighed and traipsed back towards the top of the lake. Imogen followed. She couldn't see Isaac anywhere: she couldn't even see any rockhopper penguins. This was exactly what she had been so afraid of.

'*There* you are!' said Mrs Stewart, as their parents finally caught up with them.

Mr Stewart huffed and puffed and looked put out at having to hurry.

'We can't find him,' said Imogen, in a very small voice. 'We've looked everywhere.'

'Oh, no,' said Mrs Stewart. 'Perhaps you were wrong, after all?'

'I was *not* wrong,' said Imogen crossly.

'Well, I'm sure Einstein has *other* friends back in Sydney.' Mrs Stewart crouched down and smiled at her, like she used to when Imogen was little and had been upset about something. 'So it's not the end of the world now, is it? We've still had lots of fun!'

Imogen was furious. How could her mother talk to her like that? She wasn't little, and she certainly wasn't upset – she was righteously angry. To suggest that it didn't matter that Isaac was still missing – the very idea was ridiculous!

'We did not come here,' she said through gritted teeth, 'to have *fun*!'

Mr Stewart disguised a chuckle with a fit of coughing. Then, as Imogen looked up to scold him, she saw something moving through the crowd beyond her father's shoulder: a hat, a hat with a very wide brim, and a man in a white coat attached to the bottom of it. He was passing a small building that looked like it might have offices inside, just beyond the penguin enclosure. Imogen squinted. He was about to walk inside, passing under a sign that said **Education Centre.**

'It's him!' she shouted. 'He must have Isaac!'

'It's who, dear?' said Mrs Stewart.

Imogen ignored her. 'Arthur, follow me,' she commanded.

'Imogen, Arthur! Where are you going?! Come back here!' Their mother's voice faded into the crowd as they hurried away from her.

'Excuse me!' said Imogen, in a loud and important sort of voice. 'Excuse me, sir!'

Arthur caught up with her just as the man in the white coat turned to see who was speaking to him. His face darkened. 'You,' he said.

Imogen gaped up at him, and whatever she was about to say got caught somewhere in the middle of her throat. She'd forgotten how scary he looked, with a pale, cross-looking face, and scraggly grey eyebrows that were much too big for his forehead.

'You stole my notes,' he said.

Instinctively Arthur put his hand on Imogen's

elbow, and she puffed her chest out in a renewed bout of bravery. 'And *you* stole my poster,' she retorted.

'I think we need to have a little chat,' said the man.

'So do I!' said Imogen. 'I'd like to ask you some questions!'

The man looked a little confused. 'Right, well.' He glanced around, then pointed to the nearest door. 'In here,' he said. 'After you.'

'No, after you.' Imogen folded her arms.

The man narrowed his eyes and then shrugged. 'Whichever you prefer,' he said. 'I'll be asking you the same questions either way.'

They marched into the room in a sort of procession. Einstein was still tucked safely inside Imogen's coat – she had hissed at him to stay there – and she could feel him start to wriggle impatiently.

It appeared to be some sort of cleaning cupboard. There was an old table in the centre of the room with a couple of rickety-looking chairs pulled up to it. Beyond them were several shelves of cleaning products and a disorganised selection of mops and brooms. The ceiling light was broken, occasionally giving a nervous sputter of electricity, and the blinds were pulled down.

'Sit down,' said Imogen.

The man sat down without thinking, then frowned and jumped back up again. 'Hang on,' he said, and readjusted his hat. 'Detective Bill Hunter,' he announced proudly. 'I'm looking for a penguin, and I think you might be able to help me. Perhaps you could start by telling me your name?'

'What are you doing?' Arthur whispered nervously, but Imogen hushed him.

'DCI Imogen Stewart,' she replied. 'This is my assistant, Arthur. And it just so happens that we're looking for a penguin too.' She wasn't sure what DCI stood for, but she had heard detectives say it like that on the television.

'Right,' said the man, blinking at her. 'You're a – how old are you?'

'Nine and three-quarters.'

Detective Bill Hunter shook his head. 'How can you possibly have reached that rank?'

'I'm not sure that's important right now,' said Imogen, folding her arms.

'No – I suppose not.'

'My poster,' said Imogen. 'Why did you take it down?'

'It was imperative to the operation. I believed that I recognised the penguin in question,' said Bill Hunter. 'Why did you put it up?'

'I was looking for the penguin in question.'

'Why?'

'Because the penguin in question was friends with a different penguin.' Imogen frowned: she had confused herself. 'A penguin in a different question,' she added, though she couldn't quite remember what the question was.

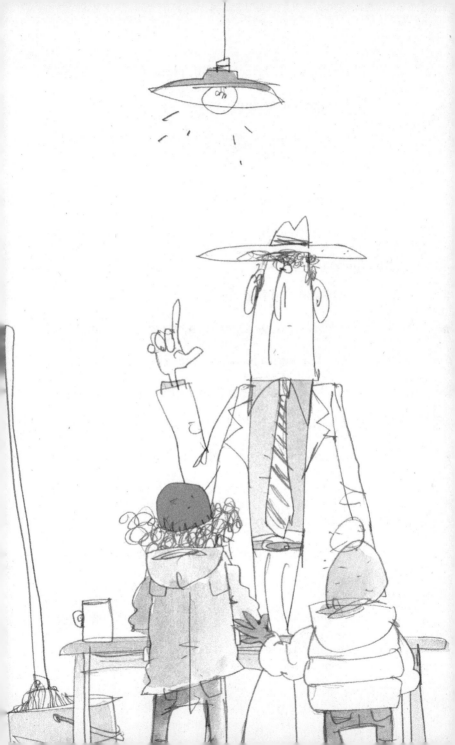

'Einstein,' said Detective Bill Hunter.

Arthur gaped at him, but Imogen kept her face deliberately blank. 'How do you know about Einstein?' she asked.

'How do *you* know about Einstein?' he shot back.

'I'm sorry,' said Imogen sarcastically. 'Who's doing the questioning here?'

'Well, I am.' Bill Hunter frowned. 'Aren't I?'

Now it was Imogen's turn to frown. 'No I am,' she said. She glanced uncertainly over at her brother.

Arthur looked at her significantly. He was thinking back to when Einstein had attacked Jack Jones in the changing rooms at school, but he was much too nervous to say anything, so tried to express the thought to her in glances.

'What?' said Imogen. She turned back to the man. 'Look, are you going to tell us where Isaac is or not?'

'No,' said Bill Hunter. He smiled menacingly. '*You*'re going to tell *me* where Einstein is, or else you'll be very, very sorry.'

'Let him out,' whispered Arthur.

Imogen's stomach did a little somersault. Detective Bill Hunter was towering above her: his hat almost blocked out the flickering ceiling light.

'Let him out of your coat,' said Arthur, more loudly this time.

Imogen did as her brother told her. She undid the top two toggles on her duffel coat and Einstein leaped out from his hiding place like a ball being launched from a very small cannon.

'Aha!' said Detective Bill Hunter triumphantly, and then, a little less triumphantly, 'Ah . . .' He took a step backwards as Einstein jumped at him, and stumbled over as he crashed into the back of one of the rickety chairs, which broke underneath his lumbering weight. He landed on the floor in a heap of wood and chair legs. His hat landed a metre or so away, revealing a mop of wiry grey hair.

'Now stop it—' he began, but he couldn't finish his sentence: Einstein was pecking his ears and tugging his hair with his beak.

Imogen took a step forward. Now *she* was towering over Detective Bill Hunter. 'Where is Isaac?' she asked.

'Get the penguin off me!'

'Have you kidnapped him? Have you murdered him?' Her eyes widened. 'Have you stuffed him and put him in a museum?'

Bill Hunter frowned. 'No, of course not, I – ow! I'm not after Isaac!'

'Einstein, wait,' said Imogen, and Einstein paused his pecking. She took another step forward. 'Who are you after, then?'

'Einstein,' said Bill Hunter. 'I've been employed by Sydney Zoo. I've traced him all the way from Australia.'

'Oh,' said Imogen awkwardly. 'And what are you going to do with him?'

'Well, I was *going* to take him home,' he said,

shooting Einstein a dirty look. 'But now I'm not sure I want to.'

'No, that's fair,' Imogen admitted. 'And . . . Isaac?'

Detective Bill Hunter shrugged. 'I knew Einstein would be looking for him.'

'We're just trying to reunite them,' Arthur piped up. 'Einstein misses his friend – he wanted to make sure he was okay. That's all. We're sorry for causing you trouble.'

Bill Hunter gave a scoffing laugh. 'I don't care what Einstein wants. Doesn't make a difference to my pay cheque.'

Imogen narrowed her eyes at him. 'You need to tell us where Isaac is so that Einstein can see him.'

'Please,' added Arthur.

'I don't and I won't!'

'Einstein, peck him!'

'All right, all right,' said Bill Hunter, shielding his face with his hands. 'He's on the other side of the path.

There's a smaller enclosure with just a few rockhopper penguins inside. Can I get my hat back?'

'You're not going to follow us, are you?' said Imogen.

Then Einstein gave a squawk, and everyone turned to look at him. He had waddled over to one of the cleaning shelves, and was attempting to pick up a roll of masking tape with his beak.

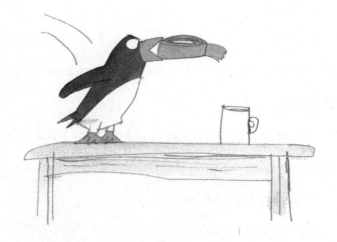

'Now look here,' Bill Hunter began. 'That really won't be necessary—'

'But we're not taking any risks,' Imogen finished,

and Einstein pecked him still while Imogen and Arthur tied him to the chair with masking tape. Then Arthur picked up a mop bucket and placed it upside down over Detective Bill Hunter's head, for good measure.

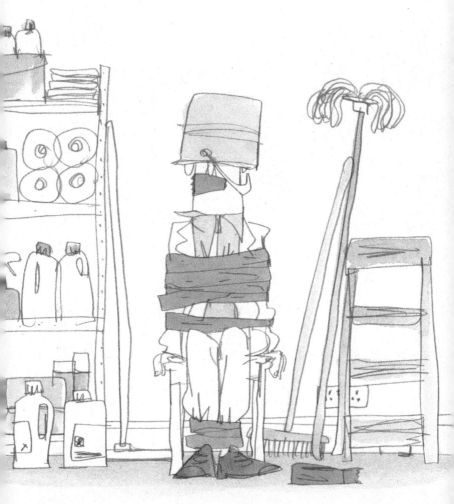

They looked at each other and smiled.

'Penguin enclosure?' said Imogen.

She scooped Einstein up off the floor and tucked him back into her coat, and Arthur followed her out of the room.

CHAPTER TWELVE

Isaac

Mr and Mrs Stewart were still waiting by the penguin enclosure when Imogen and Arthur found them. Mrs Stewart looked frantic.

'Where *have* you two been?' she said.

'Sorry,' said Imogen. They had been gone almost fifteen minutes. 'We were just investigating.'

'We know where Isaac is!' said Arthur.

Mrs Stewart's eyes flashed in anger. 'I should certainly hope you do, young man,' she said, 'after that little performance.'

'We're really very sorry,' said Imogen, 'but it was imperative to the operation.'

'It was what? Since when did you know what "imperative" means?'

Imogen shrugged.

'Your mother's right,' said Mr Stewart. 'You should never run off like that. No matter how upset you are.'

'Sorry,' said Arthur.

'It won't happen again,' Imogen added.

'So where *is* this penguin of yours?'

They led their parents over to the smaller penguin enclosure. Just as Detective Bill Hunter had said, there were the rockhopper penguins. Each one had red eyes surrounded by tufts of yellow feathers, and they were happily splashing around in the water.

'Is that him?' cried Arthur. They pushed their way to the front of the enclosure to get a better look.

'I think he's the one on the right,' said Imogen. She unbuttoned her coat slightly, to give Einstein room to

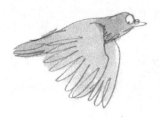

poke his head out. 'Einstein, can you see your friend?' she asked.

A barely suppressed squawk of happiness from Einstein confirmed what they already knew, but Isaac was oblivious: he couldn't see Einstein yet, and was busy watching a pigeon flap past above his head.

Imogen turned to her parents. 'He's here!' she said. 'He's the one by the rock.'

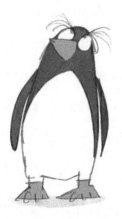

Mrs Stewart squinted. 'I don't know how you kids can tell the difference . . .' she said vaguely.

'It's Einstein!' said Imogen. 'Look at him! *He* knows!'

'Well, what now?' asked Mr Stewart.

It was a pertinent question. Arthur looked up at his sister.

'I don't know,' said Imogen. She had worried about this earlier: they had found Isaac – Einstein could see him – but what could they do about it? It was a zoo, after all, and enclosures had walls.

'You could hold Einstein up in the air and see if Isaac spots him?' suggested Mrs Stewart, filling in the silence. 'He might come over then.'

'We can't just reveal Einstein in the middle of the zoo,' said Imogen, looking at her mother as if she was an idiot. 'We'll draw attention to ourselves. They'll think we've stolen him.'

'Well, what *can* we do, then?' said Mrs Stewart, a little hurt. 'At least I'm thinking of ideas. You're all thinking of nothing but problems.'

Mr Stewart didn't appear to be thinking of problems, though. In fact, it wasn't clear *what* Mr Stewart was thinking about – only that he was thinking. His hands were in the pockets of his long coat and he was staring out into the penguin enclosure, frowning seriously. Suddenly he strode over to one of the zookeepers, adjusting his tie and straightening his collar as he walked.

'Government zoo inspection,' he said importantly. 'I'd like to take a look at one of your rockhopper penguins.'

Imogen and Arthur gaped at him.

The zookeeper looked startled. 'Oh – sorry, sir. I didn't realise we had an inspection today.'

'Your lack of organisation is none of my concern,' said Mr Stewart, checking his watch pointedly. 'But never mind. Shall we get on?'

'Erm . . . if you come into the office first, we can fill out the paperwork?'

'I'm running late for my next appointment. If we

could do it electronically afterwards, that would be fantastic.'

'I don't think we do electronic forms,' said the zookeeper, baffled.

Mr Stewart raised an eyebrow. 'Really? The system was updated three weeks ago. I'm amazed you haven't caught up with it.'

'Of course, sir. Sorry, sir,' said the zookeeper quickly. 'Which penguin was it you wanted to see?' He opened up a gate in the fence of the enclosure.

'The one by the rock,' Imogen hissed as Mr Stewart walked past.

They waited in the cold for several minutes.

'What do you think he's going to do now?' asked Arthur.

Mrs Stewart shrugged and shook her head. 'The trouble we could get into . . .' she muttered. She still wasn't over Einstein's department-store incident, and seemed twitchier than ever.

Einstein gave an anxious little squawk.

'He's right,' said Imogen, patting Einstein on the head. 'We should follow them.' Mr Stewart and the zookeeper had carried Isaac off round the corner, back towards the Education Centre.

Imogen led the way. She was just fast enough to see the back of her father's leg disappearing into an office. 'Let's listen at the window!' she said.

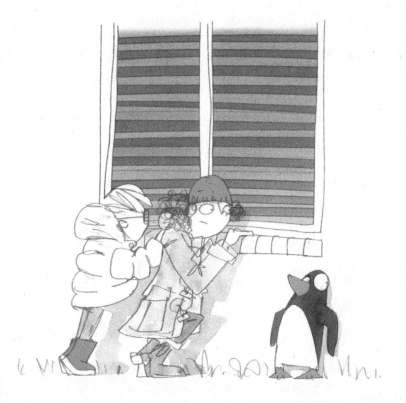

Arthur hurried after her, while Mrs Stewart – nervous about attracting attention – stuck to the path and strolled up and down it in an attempt to 'look natural'.

'Lucky they didn't go into the storage cupboard . . .' said Arthur.

They crouched down in the flowerbed beneath the office window and Imogen peeked through the blind.

'What's he *doing*?' she whispered.

As her eyes adjusted to the light, she saw Isaac standing on the desk, while a baffled-looking zookeeper watched an equally baffled-looking Mr Stewart measure his flippers with a ruler.

'Right,' said Mr Stewart. 'We'll have him back by three.'

'I'm sorry?' said the zookeeper.

Their voices were muffled through the glass, but Imogen and Arthur could just about strain to hear them.

'He's just making it up,' said Imogen.

'An Australian method,' said Mr Stewart confidently. 'We like to take the penguins out for tea once in a while, see how they're doing. Isaac's from Australia, isn't he?'

'Well, yes,' said the zookeeper. 'He came here to keep one of our other rockhoppers company. How did you know?'

'Jolly good,' said Mr Stewart, scooping Isaac up under one arm and marching purposefully towards the door while the zookeeper was still too confused to stop him.

They met on the steps outside the zoo and quickly hurried down to the pavement, where bushes shaded them from the view of the windows. Mr Stewart wiped his brow with his handkerchief and put Isaac down on the ground.

'*James!*' said Mrs Stewart, half disapproving and half impressed; and, as she didn't know which response she was going for, she was unable to follow it with anything.

Suddenly Isaac let out a gigantic honk. He stared up at Imogen's coat, where Einstein had poked his head through a gap in the buttons.

Einstein honked back.

'Oh, no,' said Mr Stewart, glancing nervously back at the zoo. 'We'd better not do this here.'

But it was too late: Imogen had placed Einstein down on the ground, and Isaac – still letting out the occasional squawk – was bouncing up and down in circles, hopping away in a state of distraction, and then hopping quickly back again to nuzzle his beak against Einstein's.

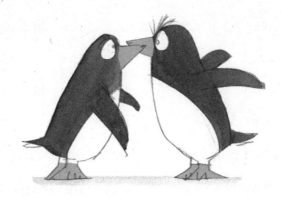

Arthur grinned, and looked ready to jump up and down too.

'Let's hail this taxi,' said Mrs Stewart, also keen to herd everyone away from the zoo.

'Can we keep Isaac as well?' said Arthur.

'I told the zookeeper I'd have him back by three,' said Mr Stewart firmly. 'But that gives us plenty of time for tea. Shall we go to the Balmoral?'

The Balmoral Hotel was very grand. Imogen thought that, from the outside, it looked like a castle or a sort of palace – somewhere that the Queen might live. The inside had chandeliers hanging from the ceiling and great big armchairs at each of the tables instead of chairs.

No one seemed to consider that they should probably have been eating lunch: it was the sort of event that called for celebration. And that meant tea and cake and scones. Arthur had a hot chocolate, but Imogen was feeling all grown up again, and insisted on sharing her parents' pot of tea. She didn't much like the tea. It was bitter, and tasted nothing like she thought it would. Mr Stewart laughed at her and filled her cup with sugar until it was drinkable.

Isaac and Einstein had an armchair too. The waiter raised an eyebrow when he saw them and whispered something to his manager, but after Mr Stewart went over and spoke to them no one seemed to say another word about it. Imogen thought Einstein looked just like royalty as he pecked at the edge of a carrot cake, and slurped up the puddle of sugary tea she had spilled on to her saucer. Isaac didn't drink any tea, but he had most of one of the pots of jam and got half of it all over the white tablecloth.

Eventually Arthur said what they had all been thinking. 'So Einstein and Isaac won't get to stay together,' he said, 'after Einstein came all this way?'

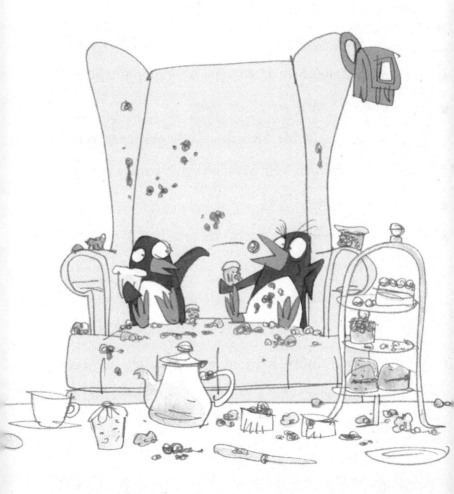

Imogen scowled at him. 'You'll upset them,' she hissed, but Einstein looked all right. The penguins had been squawking away at each other the whole way in the taxi, and Arthur had listened very hard to see if he could understand them, but whatever penguins spoke wasn't anything like English.

'Well,' said Mrs Stewart, 'he knows *where* Isaac is and that he's happy, and that's the important thing. He doesn't have to worry any more.'

'Yes,' said Mr Stewart. 'The zookeeper said he was settling in well. Led a penguin parade last week, apparently.'

Arthur liked that idea. He imagined Isaac playing the bagpipes as he headed a sort of march round the city. 'So Isaac doesn't mind living in a zoo?'

Mr Stewart looked surprised. 'Why would he mind it? He's always lived in a zoo, hasn't he? I just wonder why Sydney Zoo didn't put more effort into finding Einstein . . .'

Imogen and Arthur glanced at each other.

'You know we'll have to tell Sydney Zoo about Einstein now, don't you?' said Mrs Stewart. 'We can't keep him hidden at home forever. It wouldn't be right.'

'Yes, we knew that. It's just . . .' Imogen began. 'Aren't animals supposed to be free?'

'I suppose so,' said Mr Stewart. 'But, then again, they're not supposed to live in houses in London, either. And *we* don't exactly have a lake for them to swim in.'

'But maybe if we explain everything to the zoos,' said Arthur hopefully, 'they'll let Isaac and Einstein reunite properly?'

'Well, where there's a will there's a way,' said Mr Stewart. 'I can help you write the letter.'

'And maybe Einstein can visit us again?' added Arthur.

'He'll certainly have an open invite,' said Mrs Stewart.

Arthur supposed that that would have to do for now.

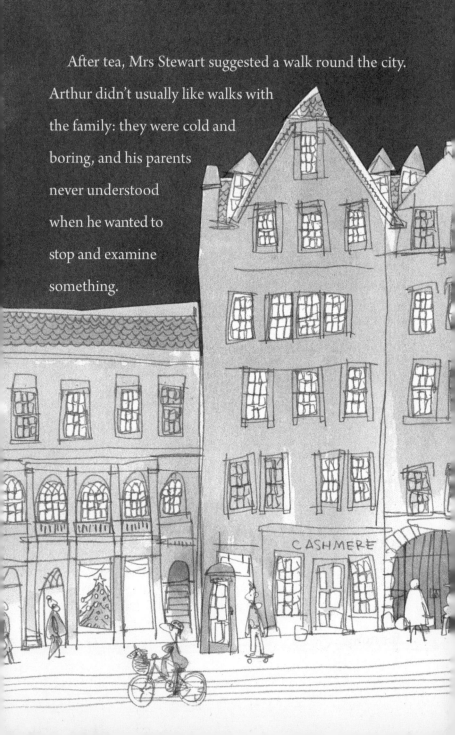

After tea, Mrs Stewart suggested a walk round the city. Arthur didn't usually like walks with the family: they were cold and boring, and his parents never understood when he wanted to stop and examine something.

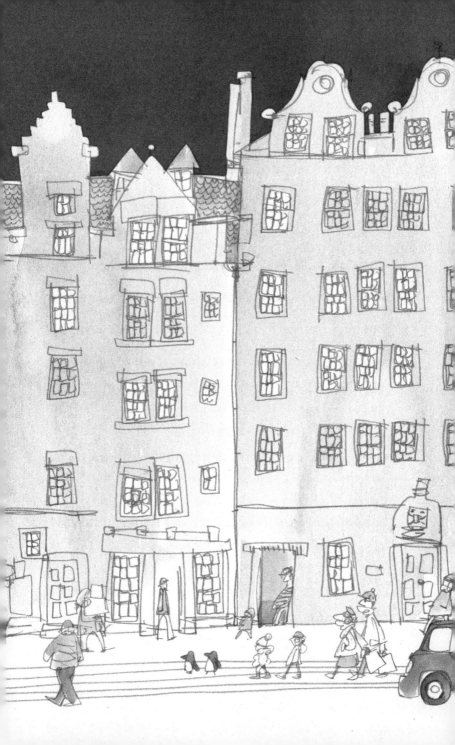

But walking round Edinburgh with two penguins was completely different. It seemed like the other pedestrians hadn't seen many penguins about, and lots of them stopped and stared, or poked each other and whispered in surprise.

Still, neither Einstein nor Isaac minded the attention, and they fluffed up their feathers with pride. Imogen didn't mind it, either, and wandered around with her head held high, as if she went for walks with penguins every day, and disapproved of anyone who didn't. The grey sky was turning white at the edges and, in the little sunlight that shone through the clouds, she felt quite sure that it was sparkling.

Even the ground beneath her feet felt different: it was firmer than usual, and somehow bouncy. The wind felt sharp and bright and the pavements smelled of rain getting ready to fall. She was a detective. She had solved her first case. And Isaac and Einstein walking side by side just a few metres away – that was all because of her.

When it was time to drop Isaac back at the zoo, everyone was exhausted.

Imogen and Arthur both hugged him goodbye, Einstein gave him a beak-nuzzle, and Mrs Stewart leaned down to say, 'Now, dear,' and used her handkerchief to wipe a lump of jam off his feathers.

'Are we ready, then?' said Mr Stewart, and he led Isaac back up the steps towards the ticket office, straightening his collar as he went.

CHAPTER THIRTEEN

Christmas

Arthur woke up early on Christmas Day, too early to go downstairs, so he looked out of his bedroom window and watched the sunrise. Grey clouds were heaving themselves awake and slouching about in the sky above the city, occasionally stopping to shimmer in a half-hearted patch of light. Down below, a pigeon was rummaging through the dustbins in the street and a pair of robins were hopping in and out of a hedge.

Just as he was wondering whether it was still too early to wake his sister, the door creaked open.

'Arthur!'

It was Imogen. She had pulled last year's Christmas jumper on over the top of her blue pyjamas, and failed to brush her hair. 'Let's go downstairs – it's Einstein's last day!'

'*And* it's Christmas,' Arthur reminded her, but this seemed somehow secondary. Arthur had spent hours and hours on Christmas Eve putting Einstein's present together, and it was that thought, more than anything, that had woken him up so early.

He followed his sister down the stairs. Somewhere behind their parents' bedroom door Mr Stewart groaned at the sound of creaking floorboards, and Imogen giggled and looked guilty.

Einstein was awake already too. Mr and Mrs

Stewart hadn't been sure, upon questioning, whether penguins celebrated Christmas, but, seeing Einstein waiting for them on the sofa downstairs, Imogen felt quite certain that they did.

'Merry Christmas, Einstein!' she cried, and dug her hand into the box of decorations to find him a Santa hat. She picked out Arthur's hat from a couple of years ago, which was much too big for Einstein's head, but when Imogen tied it back with a piece of tinsel she could just about get it to stay on. Then, in a fit of inspiration, she decided it might be nice if they woke their parents up with coffee, and had broken a mug before a minute was out.

'Do you know how to make coffee?' asked Arthur, who wanted to watch TV.

'No,' said Imogen, sweeping the broken pieces of china in the general direction of the bin. 'But I think you use coffee powder.'

She found some on the shelf and read the label while the kettle boiled. 'How many spoons do you think I should use?'

Arthur shrugged. 'Four?' he guessed.

Imogen nodded seriously. 'Maybe a few more,' she said. 'Just in case.'

She balanced the coffee very carefully on the way up the stairs, only spilling a tiny bit on to the tray. *This is going to be a very good Christmas*, she thought to herself, as she pushed open the door of her parents' bedroom.

'Merry Christmas! I brought you your coffee.'

Mr Stewart sat up in bed and rubbed his eyes. 'What time is it?'

'It's past eight,' said Imogen.

Mrs Stewart was impressed. 'Wow, well done!' she said. 'I didn't know you could make coffee.'

'Neither did I!' Imogen grinned, and Mr Stewart looked trepidatious.

All in all, Imogen was pleased

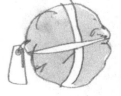

with the coffee's reception. It was just a *bit* strong, Mr Stewart had said, but not bad for a first go. Neither of them finished their cups, but then again they often didn't. Mrs Stewart placed them both back on the tray and got up to look for her dressing gown.

'It's Einstein's last day . . .' said Imogen a little sadly, though of course her parents already knew that. Mr Stewart had called Sydney Zoo as soon as they returned from Edinburgh, and the woman he spoke to on the phone had been so surprised by the story that she had quickly agreed to let Einstein stay the extra few days until Christmas.

'How funny! We sent a detective out to look for him ourselves, but we haven't heard a peep,' she had said, and then laughed. 'We'll have someone collect him from Heathrow on Boxing Day. And perhaps we'll send a few reporters too!'

Imogen liked that second idea. Maybe

Einstein would make the newspapers again and, if he did, surely *she* would too, and she'd become a world-renowned detective, and people would travel from far and wide to speak to her, and Einstein would visit every Christmas forever, and someday somebody would write a book about them . . .

Still, all that was rather a lot to wish for on just one Christmas, so she settled for a quiet, 'I hope it snows.'

'Imogen?' said Mrs Stewart, calling her out of her daydream. 'Shall we go downstairs for breakfast?'

Imogen's hopes for Christmas Day were certainly not disappointed.

It went, for the most part, like a normal Christmas, only none of the boring bits were boring any more.

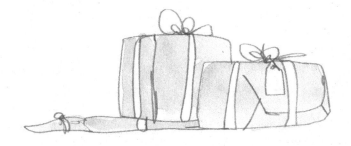

Even when Arthur had to phone his godparents to thank them for his presents – and Arthur had never liked phone calls – he could watch Einstein getting himself tangled up in tinsel on the far side of the room, and arguing with the cat over a fish-shaped toy. Sometimes, to mix things up, Imogen would hide the toy under a cushion and watch mischievously as the two animals followed each other in circles round the sofa.

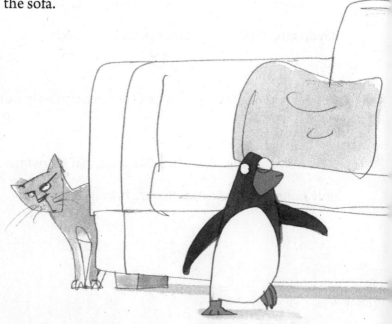

'Do you think,' said Arthur to Mrs Stewart, as Imogen distracted herself with games, 'that Theo will still want to be my friend at school?' The idea had been nagging at him ever since their trip to Edinburgh, only until now he hadn't been quite sure what it was that he was worried about.

'What do you mean, dear?' said Mrs Stewart, who was admiring the book Mr Stewart had bought her for Christmas.

'When Einstein goes home to Sydney. What if Theo doesn't like me when I don't have a penguin?'

'But Theo's only ever met Einstein once, dear,' said Mrs Stewart dismissively. 'It's not like you ever took him to school.' Then she looked suspicious.

Arthur quickly realised what he had done, and even Imogen, who had been laughing at the cat until a moment ago, turned from the sofa and looked at her brother with wide eyes.

'You didn't!' said Mrs Stewart, after a pause.

The silence answering her informed her that they did.

'I'm saying nothing,' said Mrs Stewart stiffly. She held her hands in the air and went to adjust something on the Christmas tree. 'I wish you luck if your father ever finds out!'

'Finds out what?' said Mr Stewart, who had just returned from scraping ice off the car windscreen outside.

'It wasn't me,' said Imogen quickly.

'But you *knew*!' said Arthur.

'Not at first!'

'She blackmailed me!'

'Ah,' said Mr Stewart eventually. 'Yes, I thought so. Penguins at school, hmm?'

The rest of his family looked at him in astonishment.

Mr Stewart shrugged and gave a half-smile as he hung up his coat. 'The herrings we left out were always eaten rather tidily,' he said simply. 'And Gizmo's been getting a little fat lately, don't you think?'

He wandered over to the sofa, whistled and picked up a newspaper.

'Of course Theo will still want to be your friend, Arthur,' said Imogen kindly. She was feeling a little guilty at the mention of blackmail.

'But we only made friends because of Einstein.'

'You only spoke to him because of Einstein. That's not the same thing.'

'Why don't you phone him?' suggested Mrs Stewart, who had just about recovered from her shock.

Arthur looked alarmed at the prospect.

'Go on,' said Imogen. 'You can ask him if he still wants to be friends when you wish him a happy Christmas.'

'All right . . .' said Arthur, and his stomach somersaulted as he went over to the phone.

Theo's mother picked up after a few rings.

'Merry Christmas!' Arthur mumbled, his ears going pink. 'It's Arthur. Can I speak to Theo?'

He waited for a moment while Theo came to the phone.

'Arthur!' said Theo. 'Merry Christmas!'

'Merry Christmas,' said Arthur. Then quickly, so as to get it over with: 'Einstein's going home tomorrow,' he blurted.

'Home?'

'Back to Sydney Zoo. We found Isaac, but now they want Einstein back.'

'Oh,' said Theo. 'Are you okay?'

'I think so,' said Arthur. 'Penguins aren't really meant to live in houses in London. But I hope maybe they'll let him visit.'

'Or we could go to Sydney to see him!' said Theo.

Arthur's heart lifted at that. 'So you still want to be my friend?' he said.

Theo sounded confused. 'Yes,' he said. 'Don't you?'

'Yes, of course!' said Arthur.

'Well, that's good!' said Theo. 'I need to help my

mum get dinner ready, but tell me about Isaac soon!'

'There, that wasn't so bad, was it?' said Mrs Stewart, once Arthur had put the phone down. 'Are we ready to give Einstein his Christmas presents?'

Arthur jumped up. He had been ready all day. He had painted a huge picture of Einstein and Isaac by Edinburgh Castle. Isaac's eyebrows were made of yellow pipe cleaners, his webbed feet were a string of orange fingerprints, and even Einstein's dark blue feathers were painted with a coat of glitter. It was, in everyone's opinion, his finest work to date, and the first thing to be tucked neatly into Einstein's rucksack, ready for his journey home.

Mr and Mrs Stewart had got him a framed photo of the whole family eating tea at the Balmoral Hotel. Imogen thought she looked a little silly in it, with a face full of scone, but Einstein and Isaac looked so handsome on their armchairs that she didn't really mind. And Imogen had saved him her favourite

Inspector Bucket book. She supposed that, given her success as a detective, she didn't need it so much any more, and at any rate it was something for him to remember her by. These both went in the rucksack too, along with an old scarf of Imogen's, and one of Arthur's pyjama tops. ('In case he gets cold on the flight,' Mrs Stewart explained.)

Then Imogen and Arthur opened the last of their presents, which included *more* pyjamas and *more* books, and Christmas dinner was the most delicious it had ever been, and Mr and Mrs Stewart drank rather more mulled wine than they ought to, and told Imogen off when she tried to steal some for herself.

And after more games, and Christmas crackers, and several different arguments they didn't really mean, Imogen and Arthur fell asleep in front of the telly, with the fire roaring, and Einstein snoring, and their fluffiest new Christmas socks on.

CHAPTER FOURTEEN

Goodbye For Now

Imogen woke up in her own bed, which was strange because she couldn't remember how she'd got there. There was a gentle tap on the door and Mrs Stewart stuck her head round it.

'Get dressed,' she said. 'It's time to take Einstein to the airport.'

Imogen's stomach sank a little. It hadn't seemed to matter so much a few days earlier because the excitement of Christmas had been enough to overpower any dread about Einstein going away.

But now Christmas was over, and it hadn't snowed – it was only raining, and to make matters worse the sun hadn't bothered to rise. She quickly dressed and hurried downstairs to the kitchen.

Her family was waiting in the hall and Einstein, for the first time in several weeks, was standing with his orange rucksack by the door. Mrs Stewart had wrapped a little scarf round his neck and given him a sandwich box of herrings, and he looked, to Imogen's disappointment, perfectly happy.

'Come on, everyone!' said Mr Stewart, in his cheery voice. 'Someone's got a plane to catch!'

As they climbed into the car, the sun was starting to think about coming up, but it wasn't yet bright enough for the streetlamps to have been switched off, and they lit up the falling raindrops one by one. Imogen stared out of the window as the car twisted through the streets away from their home and spotted several of her Missing Pengwin posters still hanging raggedly from walls and lamp posts. One of them had torn almost in half, and was blowing listlessly in the wind. She chewed the inside of her cheek and thought about how much younger and sillier she had been those two entire weeks ago. It was a long drive to Heathrow, and she drifted in and out of sleep for most of the way.

Heathrow Airport was busy, and once Mr Stewart had managed to park the car they had to weave through lots of groups of people to get to the check-in desk. Arthur kept hold of Einstein and was careful not to lose sight of his father's coat.

When they reached the desk, a friendly-looking flight attendant dressed in a uniform appeared to be waiting for them. She was holding a sign that read **Einstein** and recognised them before they recognised her – because they were, after all, the only family in Heathrow airport with a penguin.

'The Stewart family?' said the flight attendant. 'I'm here to escort an unaccompanied penguin.'

'That's us,' said Mr Stewart, and he shook her hand and started talking about something or other that was very important, like passport stamps and air turbulence.

Arthur and Imogen stayed a few metres behind him.

'I'll write to you,' said Arthur, putting Einstein down on the floor and giving him a hug. 'You can get one of the zookeepers to hand you the letters.'

'And maybe we'll visit Sydney?' said Imogen, glancing hopefully at her mother. 'And you can come back here whenever you like. Can't he, Mum?'

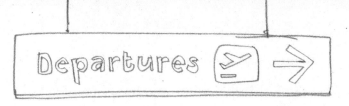

Mrs Stewart smiled. 'Of course,' she said. 'Penguins are always very welcome at our house. We'll just have to get the zoo's permission this time.'

'But if he's broken out once . . .' Arthur pointed out.

'Exactly,' said Imogen. 'It's only goodbye till we see him again.' She really meant it too. She knelt down and gave Einstein a big hug, and he squawked something that was probably along the lines of missing them both, and hoping they would visit Australia soon.

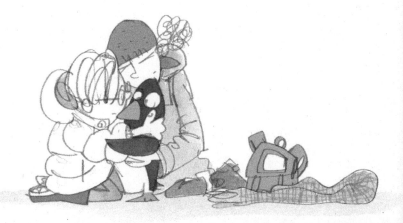

'Righto,' said Mr Stewart. 'Are we ready?'

'I think so,' said Arthur, and Imogen nodded.

'All right, Einstein,' said the flight attendant kindly. 'Would you like to come with me?'

The sinking feeling in Imogen's stomach was starting to disappear, turning into something that was still a little sad, but only in a temporary, happy sort of way. It was an odd way to feel, she thought, but not altogether a bad one. And so they watched Einstein walk through the airport, holding the flight attendant's hand in his flipper, until both had disappeared round the corner.

Epilogue

Over ten thousand miles away, a disgruntled-looking detective sat forlornly on the sofa in his boss's office. His white coat was smudged with dirt, he was badly in need of a shave and his hat was nowhere to be seen.

'You're saying a penguin pecked you, and two children locked you in a store cupboard?'

The detective shivered at the word 'penguin', and spilled a small dribble of scalding-hot coffee down his shirt.

His boss looked down at him over her glasses and started to readjust the papers on her desk.

'You don't understand . . .' the detective began. 'The penguin was out of control, and the children, they weren't like ordinary children. One of them was a Detective Chief Inspector!'

'And where did you hear *that*?' asked his boss, raising a disapproving eyebrow.

He glanced round the room, as if searching his memory for something more substantial. 'Well, she told me . . .'

'I've done my own research on the case, Bill, and I can assure you that Imogen Stewart is nothing but a Year Five student with a penchant for drama. Honestly, this is worse than the time you misplaced those crocodiles in the shopping mall.'

The detective looked glum, and said nothing.

'I could understand your difficulty that time – but a penguin? Really?'

'Penguin . . .' the detective repeated under his breath. He shivered again and stared into the middle distance.

'I've been on the phone all morning, telling Sydney Zoo why a nine-year-old can solve a case my detectives can't.'

'They tied me up,' the detective whispered. 'They put a bucket on my head . . .'

'To be honest, Bill, I'm not interested,' said his boss. 'Just get out of my office.'

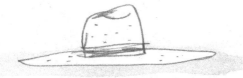

Look out for Einstein's next adventure:
THE CASE of the FISHY DETECTIVE . . .

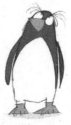

CHAPTER ONE

Back to London

Imogen was walking home from school by herself. Normally she walked with Arthur, but Arthur had gone over to Theo's house, and normally they would get the bus, but today she had missed it – and anyway, she was feeling brave.

I must look very grown up, she thought to herself, *walking along a pavement without anyone else.*

And, of course, she *was* very grown up when you thought about it. In three weeks' time she'd be eleven, and that was an impressive sort of age. Ten was double figures too, but not in such a tidy way as eleven. Eleven did double figures properly.

Imogen imagined that once she was eleven she would look and feel quite different. She would be taller and cleverer, and adults would ask her opinion on things and take her responses seriously at last. Walking home alone was simply practice for what was to come.

It was early March, and none of the trees had bothered to grow any leaves yet, so that when the wind blew, the branches looked like they were scratching the sky with their claws. But it was warm for March, and Imogen didn't mind the grey: grey was probably a sensible colour, the kind of colour she would appreciate once she was eleven.

She tucked her hands into her pockets and thought about the maths test that she had on Monday, and whether she was going to get an invite to Amy Diggory's birthday party. She didn't like the idea of not being invited, but she didn't much like the idea of going, either. It was all rather confusing to think about. And, while she'd done pretty well in her last maths test, this week Mr Smith had started putting letters into their sums, and Imogen wasn't sure whether she'd understood everything. She didn't see why numbers and letters couldn't be kept separately: when they sat next to each other like that everything went wobbly.

Still – those were problems for next week, thought Imogen, as she opened the garden gate and walked up the path towards her house. And right now it was Friday, which happened to be her favourite day of any day at all.

'It's Friday!' said Imogen, as she burst into the kitchen.

Mrs Stewart was just unpacking her work things, and Mr Stewart – who'd had the day off – was sitting with his feet up in front of the telly.

'So it is,' said Mr Stewart. 'Did they teach you that at school?'

'Can I borrow your laptop to check if the email's here?' Imogen dropped her school bag on to the floor and went to grab a biscuit from the biscuit tin.

'Just one!' said Mrs Stewart. 'And don't you want to wait until Arthur's home? He'll get upset if you open the email without him.'

'Oh,' said Imogen disappointedly. 'But what if it's important? What if Einstein's had some sort of accident, and we won't know about it because we haven't checked?'

'Those emails from Australia are the same every week,' said Mr Stewart. 'Einstein's eaten another fish and been swimming. I'm sure it can wait an hour until your brother's home.'

'It might be different this time,' said Imogen, though she didn't really mind waiting – she just liked having the last word.

'You mean he might have eaten a pilchard rather than an anchovy? Whatever will we do!' said Mr Stewart, and Imogen bounded over to the sofa to thump him with a cushion, then ran upstairs to find a book.

'Still reading about detectives?' said Mrs Stewart when she returned a moment later.

Imogen flopped down on to the sofa and sighed. 'No,' she said. 'Detectives are a bit babyish, I think.'

'Surely not!' said Mrs Stewart, aghast. 'You can't mean that.'

Imogen made a sort of mumbling noise and buried her face in her book. She didn't mean it – not really. She'd loved being a detective, and for months she'd carried her notebook with her at all times, keeping a constant eye out for things that might need investigating. But the truth was that ever since Einstein had left there hadn't been any more mysteries. Or there had – but they weren't the proper kind of mystery, the kind with heroes and villains. There were only boring mysteries: things like how to say 'hello' in French, and why Arthur never wiped his toothpaste up off the basin.

All Imogen had now to remind herself that she'd ever been a detective before were the newspaper clippings Mrs Stewart had insisted on pinning to the fridge:

Imogen Stewart:
The Girl Who Solved
The Penguin Mystery

BRITISH CHILDREN
RETURN MISSING
PENGUIN TO SYDNEY

Penguins Now Most Popular
Animals At Sydney Zoo

They were very good newspaper clippings, to be fair, and Imogen still felt a surge of pride whenever she looked at them. But it had been a whole year now – *more* than a year, in fact. It was only sensible to assume her detective days were behind her.

When Theo's mum dropped Arthur off outside the house, he was so eager to run up the path that he almost forgot to say goodbye. But he stopped himself.

'Thank you for having me!' he blurted. 'And I'll see you on Monday, Theo.'

'Are you in a rush?' Theo's mother asked.

'Oh, no,' said Arthur, going a little pink. 'But Fridays are when Ted emails us. He's the zookeeper from Sydney.'

'Ah, of course,' she said, raising her eyebrows a little. 'Silly me – how could I forget?'

Theo's mum had never actually met Einstein, and she still looked bemused whenever he was mentioned, like she didn't quite believe any of it had really happened.

'Don't worry, Mum. You'll meet Einstein next time he comes to visit,' said Theo.

'Oh, he's coming back, is he?'

'No . . . I don't know,' Arthur admitted. 'I hope so.'

'Well, tell your parents I said hello,' said Theo's mum. She'd become distracted by Theo's little sister, Sophia, who had started crying in the back seat.

Arthur waved one last time before hurrying up the garden path towards the front door.

'Imogen!' cried Arthur, as he crashed into the house and threw his school bag down on top of a pile of old trainers. 'It's Friday!'

'So it is!' called Mr Stewart. 'Did they teach you that at school?'

'That wasn't funny the first time, Dad,' said Imogen. 'Can we use the laptop now? Please?'

'Yes, yes, I demand that you use the laptop!' said Mr Stewart. 'Why haven't you used it already? This week might be the week that everything changes!'

'You're *still* not *funny!*' said Imogen, but she was already halfway up the stairs.

Dear Imogen and Arthur,

Thank you so much for your email last week! I passed everything you said on to Einstein, and he gave a very big squawk when he heard how well Arthur had done in his maths test.

This week Einstein has done a lot of swimming and has shown a preference for pilchards over anchovies. Here's a picture of him hanging out on a rock with his new friend Steve. They'd just made up after a brief incident this morning when Einstein stole Steve's fish at feeding time. I think he mostly did it because some tourists were watching. Einstein always wants to be in front of a camera . . .!

Best,

Ted

Mr Stewart had been right: it was pretty much the same as normal. But sometimes, Imogen told herself, normal was nice. It was nice knowing that Einstein was safe, and happy, and making friends with other penguins. Nine-year-old Imogen might have felt selfishly about it, and hoped for another adventure, but this Imogen – who was, after all, not so far off eleven – knew that as long as Einstein was safe everything was really all right. She smiled at the photo and started to turn away from the computer.

'Imogen, wait!' said Arthur.

'What?'

'He just sent us another message! He wants to do a video call!'

Imogen spun round. Video calls to Sydney only happened very occasionally.

Just then the desktop started to ring, and Ted's profile picture appeared above the keyboard in front of them.

Imogen rushed to click ACCEPT, and the picture expanded to fill the whole screen – only now Ted's face was moving too.

'Hi!' Ted waved, peering into the webcam.

He looked blurry at first, but eventually crackled into real time. He appeared to be in an office – the same one he'd been in last time they had spoken, in fact. Imogen couldn't remember when that was. Three weeks ago? Four?

'Can you hear me?' said Ted.

'What did he say?' whispered Arthur.

'Yes, we can hear you!' said Imogen. 'Can you see us?'

'Our camera's turned off,' said Arthur, and he elbowed Imogen out of the way to change the setting.

'Ah, there you are!' said Ted. 'How's it going?'

'Good,' said Imogen, resting her head awkwardly on her elbow. She always felt oddly shy in video calls, which was unlike her. Seeing her own miniature face in the corner made her self-conscious.

'Well, it's very late here, but I'm on the night shift so I thought I might as well let Einstein say hello.'

Arthur barged his way on to the edge of the desk chair in order to see better. Imogen was hogging it again. 'Where is he?' he asked.

'Shh,' whispered Imogen. 'Ted's *getting* him.'

They watched Ted lean down and scoop something up off the floor, and a few seconds later Einstein appeared, his feet paddling in mid-air as if he hadn't quite noticed where he was yet. Ted placed him down on the desk in front of the computer.

'Look who's here, Einstein!' said Ted.

Einstein glanced up at the screen and squawked excitedly.

'Hi, Einstein!' said Imogen.

He stretched his flippers back into the air and bounced up and down on his little feet.

'We miss you!' said Arthur. 'When are you coming back to London?'

Einstein squawked again and shrugged his flippers, then made several frantic attempts to peck the screen.

'He misses you too,' said Ted. 'Perhaps you kids could visit Sydney sometime.'

'Maybe,' said Imogen uncertainly. 'But we couldn't come alone. Mum and Dad would have to save up for it and take time off work and everything – and we don't know when that would be.'

'Yeah, it's a long way,' Ted agreed.

'We want to, though,' she added.

'You'll still let us know if Einstein ever comes to England, won't you?' asked Arthur.

'Arthur, there's no one else I would dream of telling first.'

Arthur smiled and sat back in the chair. He liked Ted. Ted always said the right thing.

'Well, I'm afraid I'm going to have to pack up in a minute, but let's talk again soon.' He ruffled Einstein's feathers and handed him a snack.

'Okay. See you soon, Einstein,' said Imogen. She brushed her finger against the screen, as if she was stroking Einstein's feathers too.

'Bye, Einstein!' said Arthur.

Einstein squawked so enthusiastically that he dropped the snack he was eating, then hurried to pick it up again and tripped over the keyboard. The picture turned the colour of feathers as Einstein came crashing towards the screen.

Imogen and Arthur heard him squawk once more before he pushed himself up with his flippers and accidentally ended the call with the edge of his beak.

To be continued…

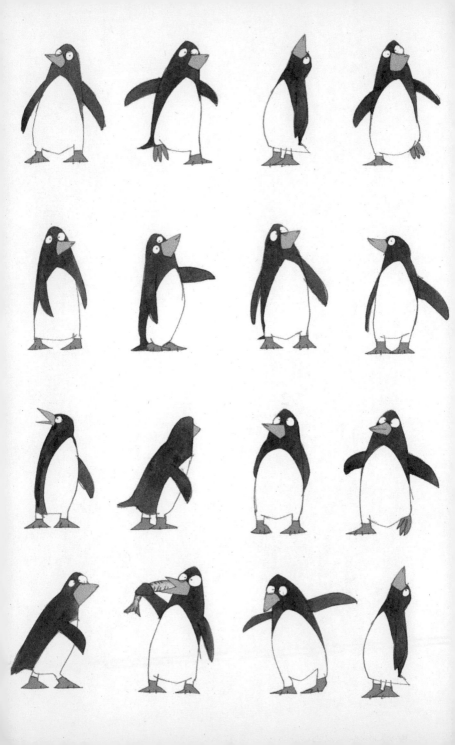

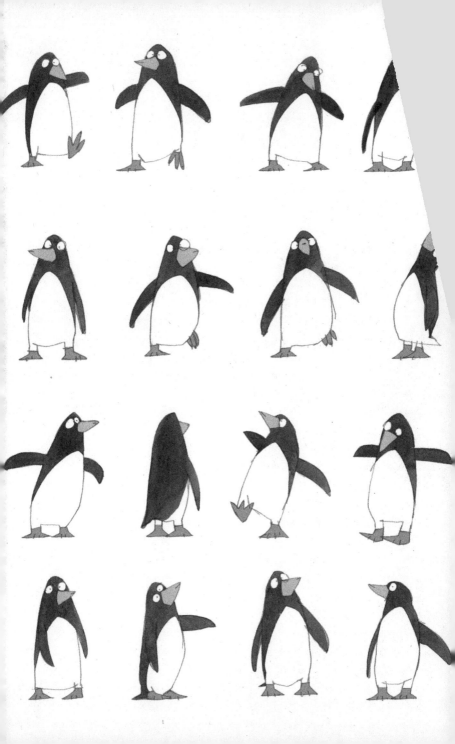